Urinary Tract Infections - New Insights
http://dx.doi.org/10.5772/intechopen.101017
Edited by Wael Hegazy

Assistants to the Editor: Azza Abdel Fatah Hassan Rajab and Lwanyumba Joram Lwegasila

Contributors
Benyamin Djawadi, Nazila Heideri, Mojtaba Mohseni, Tsegaye Melaku Kebede, Juan Xicohtencatl-Cortes, Ariadnna Cruz-Córdova, Marco A. Antonio Flores-Oropeza, Sara A. Ochoa, Rigoberto Hernández-Cruz, Guadalupe Aguirre Avalos, Gerardo Amaya-Tapia, Gabriela Ibarra-Nieto, Octavio Campollo Rivas, José Luis González Sánchez, Victor Hugo Mosquera, Wael Hegazy

First published in London, United Kingdom, 2023 by IntechOpen
IntechOpen is the global imprint of INTECHOPEN LIMITED, registered in England and Wales, registration number: 11086078, 5 Princes Gate Court, London, SW7 2QJ, United Kingdom

British Library Cataloguing-in-Publication Data
A catalogue record for this book is available from the British Library

Additional hard and PDF copies can be obtained from orders@intechopen.com

Urinary Tract Infections - New Insights
Edited by Wael Hegazy
p. cm.
Print ISBN 978-1-83769-988-9
Online ISBN 978-1-83768-212-6
eBook (PDF) ISBN 978-1-83768-213-3

For EU product safety concerns:
IN TECH d.o.o., Prolaz Marije Krucifikse Kozulić 3, 51000 Rijeka, Croatia,
info@intechopen.com or visit our website at intechopen.com.

Meet the editor

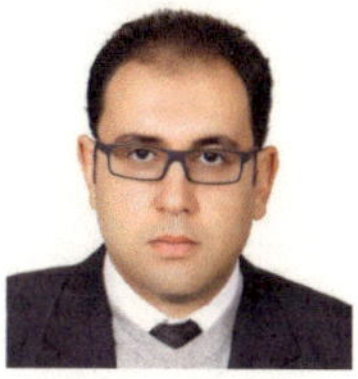

Dr. Wael A. H. Hegazy, Ph.D., is a distinguished Professor of Microbiology and Immunology, renowned for his groundbreaking research and contributions to the field. Educated at reputable institutions, Dr. Hegazy obtained his Ph.D. in Microbiology from the University of Osnabrück, Germany, where he delved into the intricate world of host–pathogen interactions. His groundbreaking doctoral research on the optimization of *Salmonella* as a carrier for cancer vaccines earned him international recognition. Throughout his extensive research journey, Dr. Hegazy has led numerous pivotal studies investigating the complex dynamics between pathogens and the immune system, and how to conquer bacterial resistance. His research publications have appeared in top-tier scientific journals, and he has authored several influential book chapters.

Contents

Preface

Welcome to the world of urinary tract infections (UTIs), a common and often underestimated health concern affecting millions of individuals worldwide. Whether you are personally dealing with UTIs or seeking knowledge to support a loved one, this book is designed to be your trusted companion in navigating the intricate landscape of UTIs.

UTIs can be a source of discomfort, frustration, and even anxiety for those who experience them. They can disrupt daily life, strain relationships, and create a sense of helplessness. However, armed with the right information and empowered by proactive strategies, you can take control of your urinary health and break free from the cycle of recurring infections.

In this book, we provide a comprehensive understanding of UTIs, including their causes, symptoms, treatments, and preventive measures. You will discover the underlying mechanisms at play within the urinary system, gaining insights that will help you demystify the complexities of this condition. We have compiled the latest medical research, expert advice, and real-life experiences to offer you a holistic perspective.

It is our sincere hope that this book will serve as a valuable resource, offering both guidance and reassurance to those seeking solutions for UTIs. Whether you are a healthcare professional, a patient, or a concerned family member, we invite you to embark on this journey of knowledge, understanding, and empowerment.

With warm regards,

Wael Hegazy
Faculty of Pharmacy,
Department of Microbiology and Immunology,
Zagazig University,
Zagazig, Egypt

Section 1

Introduction

Chapter 1

Introductory Chapter: Urinary Tract Infections (UTIs)

Wael Hegazy

1. Introduction

Urinary tract infections (UTIs) are a prevalent bacterial infection in humans, accounting for about 40% of all hospital-acquired infections [1, 2]. The occurrence of UTIs has increased by 60% in the last three decades between 1990 and 2019, highlighting the significant public health issue they pose [3]. The UTIs symptoms commonly include bacteriuria along with suprapubic discomfort, urgency, urinary frequency, and dysuria [4]. UTIs are classified into two types: uncomplicated UTIs, also known as cystitis, affect only the bladder and can be resolved with simple antibiotic treatments. While the disseminated infections to the upper urinary tract are referred as complicated UTIs, that require more aggressive antibiotic treatments for longer periods. Furthermore, complicated UTIs are associated with higher rates of sepsis, recurrent infection, treatment failure, and significant morbidity and mortality [4–7]. Uncomplicated UTIs affect 40–60% of females, at least once in their lifetime, on the other hand, all UTIs in males are usually considered complicated [8–10]. Recurrent UTIs are characterized by the occurrence of at least two acute UTI episodes within a span of 10 months or three episodes within a 12-month period, with a higher incidence in females than males [11, 12]. The UTIs can be self-infected, community-acquired, or nosocomial. Community-acquired infections typically result from low sanitary precautions, poor personal hygiene, or multiple sexual partners [7, 11]. The risk of self-infections often occurs in immunocompromised individuals as commensal inhabitants from the periurethral, vaginal, or rectal flora usually cause it [13, 14].

2. Risk factors

However, UTIs are recurrently encountered in healthcare amenities, the high infection rates could be associated with some risk factors. The gender, females are usually at high risk; it is expected that 40–60% of females will get UTIs at least once in their life, and half of them will suffer from recurrency within 1 year [9, 11, 12]. In males, the incidence of UTIs is lower than in females (10–15%), and even lower in circumcised males [10].

Females are at a higher risk of UTIs for various reasons; first of all, their shorter urethra eases the spread of bacteria to the bladder establishing infection [15]. Additionally, anatomical differences between males and females make self-infection from perineal flora more likely in females [9]. Hormonal changes during menopause, which reduce estrogen levels, also increase the risk of infection by making urogenital skin thinner and reducing the presence of protective *Lactobacilli*, as the lactic acid production by *Lactobacilli* renders the vaginal pH more acidic that does not encourage the growth of invading bacteria conferring a protective barrier against pathogenic infections [16]. Furthermore, the immunocompromised individuals including geriatrics and pregnant women are at high risk [17–20]. In diabetic patients, nephropathy, glycosuria, and reduced immunity contribute to the higher incidence of complicated UTIs [3, 21–23]. Other factors that increase the risk of UTIs comprise anatomical abnormalities of the urinary tract, kidney stones, and the use of physical interventions such as spermicides, contraceptive diaphragms, intrauterine devices, catheters, and frequent pelvic examinations [10, 14].

3. Bacterial and fungal etiology of UTIs

The bacterial etiology of UTIs involves a variety of Gram-positive and -negative bacteria as well as the most common fungal infections by *Candida* spp., mainly *C. albicans* (**Figure 1**) [2]. Typically, the infections are mostly originated from the normal flora of the urogenital system, vaginal, and rectum besides the intestinal microbiota serving as the main reservoir of infections [4, 9]. *Escherichia coli* is the most frequently identified urinary tract pathogen, responsible for 65% of complicated UTIs and 75% of uncomplicated UTIs [24]. *Klebsiella pneumoniae* is the second most frequent cause of UTIs, accounting for 6–8% of cases, while *C. albicans* and *Enterococcus faecalis* are significant causes of complicated UTIs, causing 7% and 11% of UTIs, respectively [14]. Other less commonly identified causative agents include *Staphylococcus saprophyticus*, *Staphylococcus aureus*, *Staphylococcus epidermidis*, group B *Streptococcus*, *Proteus mirabilis*, *Acinetobacter baumannii*, and *Pseudomonas aeruginosa* [14, 25].

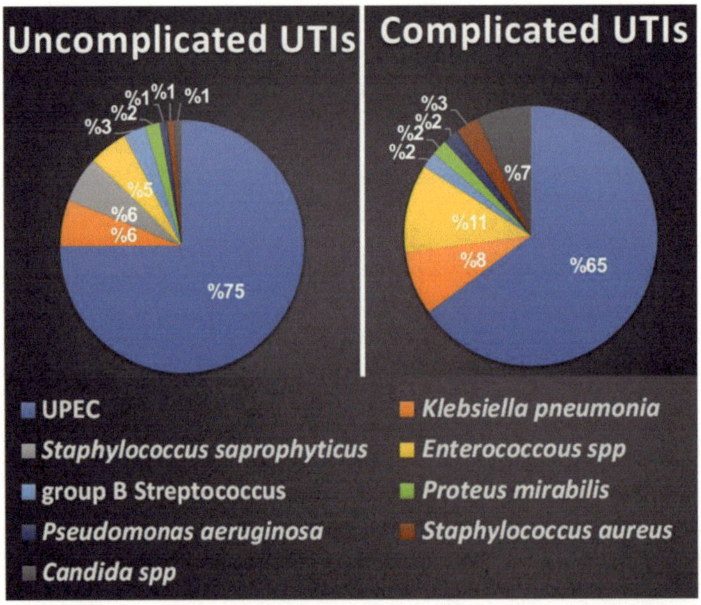

Figure 1.
The most common uropathogens (adopted from Lila et al. [2]). UTIs are caused by a wide range of Gram-positive and -negative bacterial pathogens and fungal pathogens mainly Candida spp.

4. Pathogenesis of UTIs

The bacterial ability to breach the urethral sphincter muscle, the natural barrier against pathogens, initiates pathogenesis employing bacterial fimbriae and adhesin to adhere to the urethral epithelium [26, 27]. Then, bacteria ascend the urethra and colonize the urinary bladder, where they express numerous virulence factors that promote necrosis of tissues and facilitate invasion, resulting in cystitis [4, 14, 28]. UTIs symptoms extend to include fever, suprapubic pain, lower abdominal pain, blisters, and ulcers in the urogenital area besides bacteriuria, dysuria, urgency, urinary frequency, pyuria, itching, and burning sensation during urination [29, 30].

5. Catheter-associated urinary tract infections (CAUTIs)

CAUTIs are the most frequent hospital-acquired infections and account for nearly 40% of all infections [3, 21]. Urinary catheters are foreign bodies that induce local mechanical stress, causing various inflammatory responses such as mucosal lesions edema, and exfoliation [21]. Insufficient use of aseptic techniques while inserting a catheter can cause contamination, which in turn can result in CAUTIs. The probability of developing UTIs is notably high when catheterization is prolonged (beyond 7 days) because the surface of urinary catheters provides an optimal environment for bacterial growth and attachment [21, 31]. Additionally, the deposited fibrinogen lubricates the catheter surface and serves as a nutrient source providing an ideal niche for bacterial attachment [23].

6. Biofilm formation

Biofilm formation constitutes the cornerstone in the UTIs pathogenesis playing the main role in CAUTIs [32–34]. Moreover, the formation of biofilms is regarded as a crucial factor contributing to the frequent recurrence of UTIs. In Refs. [23, 32], and antimicrobial resistance [34–37]. These biofilms are anchored in the place by an extracellular polymer matrix that is secreted by the bacteria themselves, which constitute an obstacle against antibiotics to attack bacteria [2, 26, 38]. The behavior of bacteria in biofilms is different from that of planktonic bacteria, they prioritize fortifying their establishment plan over motility and metabolic activities to conserve nutrients and energy [26, 39, 40]. They upregulate extracellular toxins to cause maximum tissue damage, releasing nutrients and cementing the biofilm in place [41, 42]. The biofilm sheds daughter planktonic cells that persistently disseminate the infection and create new biofilms. These biofilms are difficult to eradicate and can lead to chronic and recurrent infections [13, 26].

7. Objectives of UTIs book

UTIs are a common health issue that affects millions of people around the world every year, resulting in discomfort and pain that have a significant impact on a person's quality of life, and if left untreated, can lead to more serious complications. This book aims to provide a comprehensive guide to understanding UTIs, their causes, symptoms, and treatment options. Through this book, readers will gain a better understanding of the risk factors associated with UTIs, as well as ways to prevent and manage them. The book will cover both conventional and alternative treatments, as well as lifestyle changes that can help prevent UTIs from occurring. In addition to providing valuable information for those who have already experienced UTIs, this book will also serve as a valuable resource for healthcare professionals who treat patients with UTIs. By presenting the latest research and evidence-based recommendations, this book will help healthcare providers make informed decisions about diagnosis and treatment.

Author details

Wael Hegazy
Zagazig University, Zagazig, Egypt

*Address all correspondence to: waelmhegazy@daad-alumni.de

References

[1] Saint S, Kowalski CP, Kaufman SR, Hofer TP, Kauffman CA, Olmsted RN, et al. Preventing hospital-acquired urinary tract infection in the United States: A national study. Clinical Infectious Diseases: An Official Publication of the Infectious Diseases Society of America. 2008;**46**(2):243-250. DOI: 10.1086/524662

[2] Lila ASA, Rajab AA, Abdallah MH, Rizvi SMD, Moin A, Khafagy E-S, et al. Biofilm lifestyle in recurrent urinary tract infections. Life. 2023;**13**(1):148

[3] Oumer Y, Regasa Dadi B, Seid M, Biresaw G, Manilal A. Catheter-associated urinary tract infection: Incidence, associated factors and drug resistance patterns of bacterial isolates in southern Ethiopia. Infectious Drug Resistances. 2021;**14**:2883-2894. DOI: 10.2147/IDR.S311229

[4] McLellan LK, Hunstad DA. Urinary tract infection: Pathogenesis and outlook. Trends in Molecular Medicine. 2016;**22**(11):946-957. DOI: 10.1016/j.molmed.2016.09.003

[5] Medina-Polo J, Naber KG, Bjerklund Johansen TE. Healthcare-associated urinary tract infections in urology. GMS Infectious Diseases. 2021;**9**:Doc05. DOI: 10.3205/id000074

[6] Ronald A. The etiology of urinary tract infection: Traditional and emerging pathogens. The American Journal of Medicine. 2002;**113**(Suppl 1A):14S-19S. DOI: 10.1016/s0002-9343(02)01055-0

[7] Sabih A, Leslie SW. Complicated Urinary Tract Infections. Treasure Island, FL: StatPearls; 2022

[8] Medina M, Castillo-Pino E. An introduction to the epidemiology and burden of urinary tract infections. Therapeutic Advances in Urology. 2019;**11**:1756287219832172. DOI: 10.1177/1756287219832172

[9] Minardi D, d'Anzeo G, Cantoro D, Conti A, Muzzonigro G. Urinary tract infections in women: Etiology and treatment options. International Journal of General Medicine. 2011;**4**:333-343. DOI: 10.2147/IJGM.S11767

[10] Bono MJ, Leslie SW, Reygaert WC. Urinary Tract Infection. Treasure Island, FL: StatPearls; 2022

[11] Suskind AM, Saigal CS, Hanley JM, Lai J, Setodji CM, Clemens JQ, et al. Incidence and management of uncomplicated recurrent urinary tract infections in a national sample of women in the United States. Urology. 2016;**90**:50-55. DOI: 10.1016/j.urology.2015.11.051

[12] Dason S, Dason JT, Kapoor A. Guidelines for the diagnosis and management of recurrent urinary tract infection in women. Canadian Urological Association Journal. 2011;**5**(5):316-322. DOI: 10.5489/cuaj.11214

[13] Vestby LK, Grønseth T, Simm R, Nesse LL. Bacterial biofilm and its role in the pathogenesis of disease. Antibiotics (Basel). 3 Feb 2020;**9**(2):59. DOI: 10.3390/antibiotics9020059. PMID: 32028684; PMCID: PMC7167820

[14] Flores-Mireles AL, Walker JN, Caparon M, Hultgren SJ. Urinary tract infections: Epidemiology, mechanisms of infection and treatment options. Nature Reviews. Microbiology. 2015;**13**(5):269-284. DOI: 10.1038/nrmicro3432

[15] Barber AE, Norton JP, Wiles TJ, Mulvey MA. Strengths and limitations

of model systems for the study of urinary tract infections and related pathologies. Microbiology and Molecular Biology Reviews. 2016;**80**(2):351-367. DOI: 10.1128/MMBR.00067-15

[16] Storme O, Tiran Saucedo J, Garcia-Mora A, Dehesa-Davila M, Naber KG. Risk factors and predisposing conditions for urinary tract infection. Therapeutic Advances in Urology. 2019;**11**:1756287218814382. DOI: 10.1177/1756287218814382

[17] Glover M, Moreira CG, Sperandio V, Zimmern P. Recurrent urinary tract infections in healthy and nonpregnant women. Urological Science. 2014;**25**(1):1-8. DOI: 10.1016/j.urols.2013.11.007

[18] Giannakopoulos X, Sakkas H, Ragos V, Tsiambas E, Bozidis P, et al. Impact of enterococcal urinary tract infections in immunocompromised - neoplastic patients. Journal of BUON. 2019;**24**(5):1768-1775

[19] Askoura M, Abbas HA, Al Sadoun H, Abdulaal WH, Abu Lila AS, Almansour K, et al. Elevated levels of IL-33, IL-17 and IL-25 indicate the progression from chronicity to hepatocellular carcinoma in hepatitis C virus patients. Pathogens. 2022;**11**(1):57. DOI: 10.3390/pathogens11010057

[20] Hegazy WAH, Henaway M. Hepatitis C virus pathogenesis: Serum IL-33 level indicates liver damage. African Journal of Microbiology Research. 2015;**9**(20):1386-1393. DOI: 10.5897/AJMR2015.7496

[21] Venkataraman R, Yadav U. Catheter-associated urinary tract infection: An overview. Journal of Basic and Clinical Physiology and Pharmacology. 29 Aug 2022;**34**(1):5-10. DOI: 10.1515/jbcpp-2022-0152. PMID: 36036578

[22] Hegazy WAH, Rajab AAH, Abu Lila AS, Abbas HA. Anti-diabetics and antimicrobials: Harmony of mutual interplay. World Journal of Diabetes. 2021;**12**(11):1832-1855. DOI: 10.4239/wjd.v12.i11.1832

[23] Niveditha S, Pramodhini S, Umadevi S, Kumar S, Stephen S. The isolation and the biofilm formation of uropathogens in the patients with catheter associated urinary tract infections (UTIs). Journal of Clinical and Diagnostic Research. 2012;**6**(9):1478-1482. DOI: 10.7860/JCDR/2012/4367.2537

[24] Sarowska J, Futoma-Koloch B, Jama-Kmiecik A, Frej-Madrzak M, Ksiazczyk M, Bugla-Ploskonska G, et al. Virulence factors, prevalence and potential transmission of extraintestinal pathogenic *Escherichia coli* isolated from different sources: Recent reports. Gut Pathogens. 2019;**11**:10. DOI: 10.1186/s13099-019-0290-0

[25] Pinault L, Chabriere E, Raoult D, Fenollar F. Direct identification of pathogens in urine by use of a specific matrix-assisted laser desorption ionization-time of flight spectrum database. Journal of Clinical Microbiology. 28 Mar 2019;**57**(4):e01678-18. DOI: 10.1128/JCM.01678-18. PMID: 30700506; PMCID: PMC6440795

[26] Delcaru C, Alexandru I, Podgoreanu P, Grosu M, Stavropoulos E, Chifiriuc MC, et al. Microbial biofilms in urinary tract infections and prostatitis: Etiology, pathogenicity, and combating strategies. Pathogens. 30 Nov 2016;**5**(4):65. DOI: 10.3390/pathogens5040065. PMID: 27916925; PMCID: PMC5198165

[27] Askoura M, Almalki AJ, Lila ASA, Almansour K, Alshammari F, Khafagy E-S, et al. Alteration of salmonella enterica virulence and host pathogenesis through targeting sdiA by using the CRISPR-Cas9 system. Microorganisms.

2021;**9**(12):2564. DOI: 10.3390/microorganisms9122564

[28] Flores-Mireles AL, Walker JN, Bauman TM, Potretzke AM, et al. Fibrinogen release and deposition on urinary catheters placed during urological procedures. The Journal of Urology. 2016;**196**(2):416-421. DOI: 10.1016/j.juro.2016.01.100

[29] Cortes-Penfield NW, Trautner BW, Jump RLP. Urinary tract infection and asymptomatic bacteriuria in older adults. Infectious Disease Clinics of North America. 2017;**31**(4):673-688. DOI: 10.1016/j.idc.2017.07.002

[30] Chu CM, Lowder JL. Diagnosis and treatment of urinary tract infections across age groups. American Journal of Obstetrics and Gynecology. 2018;**219**(1):40-51. DOI: 10.1016/j.ajog.2017.12.231

[31] Guiton PS, Hannan TJ, Ford B, Caparon MG, Hultgren SJ. Enterococcus faecalis overcomes foreign body-mediated inflammation to establish urinary tract infections. Infection and Immunity. 2013;**81**(1):329-339. DOI: 10.1128/IAI.00856-12

[32] Rishpana MS, Kabbin JS. Candiduria in catheter associated urinary tract infection with special reference to biofilm production. Journal of Clinical and Diagnostic Research. 2015;**9**(10):DC11. DOI: 10.7860/JCDR/2015/13910.6690

[33] Balestrino D, Souweine B, Charbonnel N, Lautrette A, Aumeran C, Traore O, et al. Eradication of microorganisms embedded in biofilm by an ethanol-based catheter lock solution. Nephrology, Dialysis, Transplantation. 2009;**24**(10):3204-3209. DOI: 10.1093/ndt/gfp187

[34] Cavalu S, Elbaramawi SS, Eissa AG, Radwan MF, et al. Characterization of the anti-biofilm and anti-quorum sensing activities of the β-Adrenoreceptor antagonist atenolol against gram-negative bacterial pathogens. International Journal of Molecular Sciences. 2022;**23**(21):13088. DOI: 10.3390/ijms232113088

[35] Thabit AK, Eljaaly K, Zawawi A, Ibrahim TS, Eissa AG, Elbaramawi SS, et al. Muting bacterial communication: Evaluation of Prazosin anti-quorum sensing activities against gram-negative bacteria *Pseudomonas aeruginosa*, *Proteus mirabilis*, and *Serratia marcescens*. Biology (Basel). 2022;**11**(9). DOI: 10.3390/biology11091349

[36] Khayyat AN, Abbas HA, Khayat MT, Shaldam MA, Askoura M, Asfour HZ, et al. Secnidazole is a promising imidazole mitigator of *Serratia marcescens* virulence. Microorganisms. 2021;**9**(11):2333. DOI: 10.3390/microorganisms9112333

[37] Almalki AJ, Ibrahim TS, Elhady SS, Hegazy WAH, Darwish KM. Computational and biological evaluation of β-Adrenoreceptor blockers as promising bacterial anti-virulence agents. Pharmaceuticals. 2022;**15**(2):110. DOI: 10.3390/ph15020110

[38] Elfaky MA, Thabit AK, Eljaaly K, Zawawi A, Abdelkhalek AS, Almalki AJ, et al. Controlling of bacterial virulence: Evaluation of anti-virulence activities of Prazosin against *Salmonella enterica*. Antibiotics (Basel). 9 Nov 2022;**11**(11):1585. DOI: 10.3390/antibiotics11111585. PMID: 36358239; PMCID: PMC9686722

[39] Donlan RM, Costerton JW. Biofilms: Survival mechanisms of clinically relevant microorganisms. Clinical Microbiology Reviews. 2002;**15**(2):167-193. DOI: 10.1128/CMR.15.2.167-193.2002

[40] Khayyat AN, Abbas HA, Mohamed MFA, Asfour HZ, Khayat MT,

Ibrahim TS, et al. Not only antimicrobial: Metronidazole mitigates the virulence of *Proteus mirabilis* isolated from macerated diabetic foot ulcer. Applied Sciences. 2021;**11**(15):6847. DOI: 10.3390/app11156847

[41] Solano C, Echeverz M, Lasa I. Biofilm dispersion and quorum sensing. Current Opinion in Microbiology. 2014;**18**:96-104. DOI: 10.1016/j.mib.2014.02.008

[42] Hegazy WAH, Salem IM, Alotaibi HF, Khafagy E-S, Ibrahim D. Terazosin interferes with quorum sensing and type three secretion system and diminishes the bacterial espionage to mitigate the *Salmonella typhimurium* pathogenesis. Antibiotics. 2022;**11**:465. DOI: 10.3390/antibiotics11040465

Section 2

Urinary Tract Infections

Chapter 2

UTI Caused by *Staphylococcus saprophyticus*

Benyamin Djawadi, Nazila Heidari and Mojtaba Mohseni

Abstract

Coagulase-negative Staphylococci (CoNS) are one of the most frequently isolated bacteria in the clinical microbiology laboratory. These bacteria are normal inhabitants of human skin and mucous membranes; also, they have emerged as significant nosocomial pathogens. *Staphylococcus saprophyticus* is a Gram-positive bacterium well known for causing uncomplicated urinary tract infections in young sexually active females, responsible for complications including urinary tract infections, epididymitis, prostatitis, and acute pyelonephritis. CoNS can be divided into two groups based on susceptibility to novobiocin. The novobiocin-susceptible species include *S. epidermidis*, *S. haemolyticus*, *S. hominins*, *S. lugdunensis*, *S. schleiferi*, and the novobiocin-resistance species, including *S. saprophyticus* and *S. xylosus*. The acute uncomplicated UTI, including cystitis and pyelonephritis, is frequent in an immunocompetent nonpregnant female population, the second most common cause of community-acquired urinary tract bacterial infection in women after the *Escherichia coli*. *S. saprophyticus* is a part of the normal human flora which colonizes the rectum, urethra, cervix, and gastrointestinal tract. Bacterial colonization of the bladder and ureter epithelium occurs via several types of adhesin, including hemagglutinins with autolytic properties. Also, some strains can create and produce biofilms to increase their pathogenicity.

Keywords: *Staphylococcus saprophyticus*, UTI, coagulase-negative staphylococci, *S. saprophyticus*, CoNS, urinary tract infections

1. Introduction

Staphylococcus organisms can be coagulase-positive or negative, and Coagulase-negative Staphylococcus microorganisms are associated with human infections. *S. saprophyticus* is a clustering Gram-positive Commensal CoNS (Coagulase-negative Staphylococci), non-motile, non-spore, non-hemolytic coccus and Novobiocin-resistant which is a common urinary tract pathogen accounting for 10–20% of cases in young women, rarely associated with urinary tract infections in male populations, with the cell membrane that's made up of the typical lipid-protein bilayer made of phospholipids and the cell wall which is composed of peptidoglycan and teichoic acid that function to maintain the shape of the cell associated with adhesions, unique adhesion protein which allows it to attach to human uroepithelial cells and abundant transporter systems to adapt to changing pH and osmolarity [1]. *S. saprophyticus* is a common cause of urinary tract infections in the young, sexually active female population. There are multiple chances of developing prostatitis and urethritis in immunocompetent hosts. *S. saprophyticus* can be differentiated from other coagulase-negative Staphylococcus by its resistance to Novobiocin, and like other uropathogens, *S. saprophyticus* can produce ammonia by utilizing urease [2]. Coagulase-negative Staphylococcus can be found on the skin, rectum, urethra, and cervix as a microbiome [3–5]. *S. saprophyticus* is the second most common cause of UTI after *E. coli*. Over 40% of all sexually active females contain *S. saprophyticus* as part of their normal genitourinary flora [3–5]. General risk factors for UTIs are recent sexual intercourse, benign prostatic, pregnancy, and female sex [6]. This bacterium can encode different transport proteins, enabling it to adjust to environmental pH changes and proliferate urine.

2. Definition of UTI

Urinary tract infection, also called UTI, is one of the most common bacterial infections; it is characterized into different groups: young women with uncomplicated cystitis, female with recurrent cystitis, women with acute uncomplicated pyelonephritis, asymptomatic bacteriuria, and adults with cystitis complications. A complicated UTI is a condition that increases the risk of developing severe complications like treatment failure (**Figure 1**) [7].

UTI is a term to explain any urinary tract infection that concludes with asymptomatic bacteriuria, pyelonephritis, and cystitis. Acute complicated UTIs are typically between 27 to 44% of the healthy female with normal urinary tracts. The incidence of symptomatic UTI in men younger than 50 years is much lower than in women [8]. Asymptomatic bacteriuria is found in 5% of young women and rarely in men younger than 50 [9]. Most uncomplicated UTIs in the healthy female population has resulted from uropathogenic, found in rectal flora in men; colonizing uropathogens may also come from the partner's vagina or rectum [10]. Factors predisposing patients to develop complicated UTIs are generally caused by urine flow which facilitates the

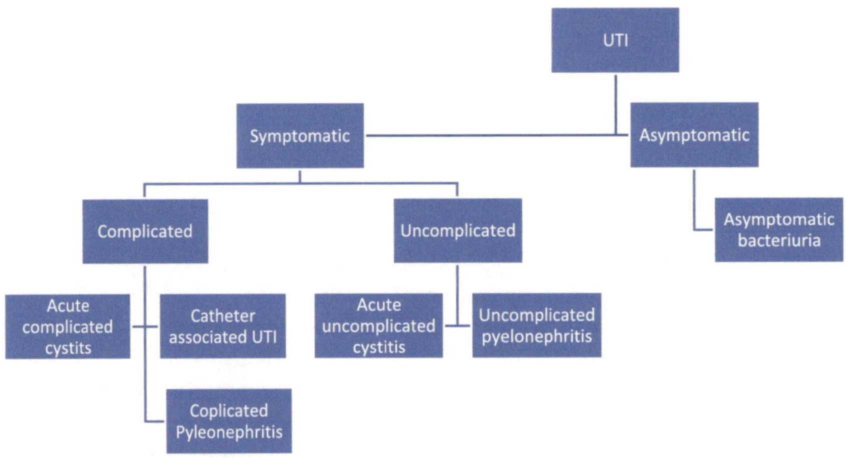

Figure 1.
Classification of UTIs in young women.

Type of Infection	Risk Factors
Premenopausal women	Having recently had sexual intercourse, Previous UTI history.
Postmenopausal women	History of previous UTI, Incomplete bladder emptying
Recurrent UTI	Recent sexual intercourse, Spermicide use, Diabetes
Pyelonephritis	Sexual intercourse, Mother with UTIs.

Table 1.
Risk factors for common UTIs.

entry of uropathogenic into the urinary tract by bypassing the host defense system [11]. Recurrent types of cystitis in healthy female is triggered when an infection is repeated during different period, which is caused by the persistence of the infected strain in the fecal flora [12]. Asymptomatic bacteriuria occurs in patients without any urinary infections [13]. Both pyelonephritis and cystitis are UTIs involving the bladder and kidneys; based on the risk factors such as gender and having sexual intercourse, other complications can be classified into complicated or uncomplicated UTIs [14]. These classifications are made to help patients in need of diagnostic tests or even more extended periods of antimicrobial treatments. On the other hand, an uncomplicated UTI can occur in a healthy nonpregnant woman with beneficial flora and no history of bladder compilations such as bladder catheterization [15]. Diabetic women are classified as a group having complicated infections. As mentioned before, cystitis and pyelonephritis are depended on the patient's risk factors, such as UTI history, diabetes, age, e, and gender. Although cystitis can progress to hostile stages and cause acute pyelonephritis, the occurrence is rare [16]. Acute pyelonephritis includes sepsis, kidney infection, and perinephric abscess [17]. Recurrent UTIs are commonly defined as infections within 12 months or predisposition to two disorders within 6 months [18]. Females diagnosed with UTI will develop a recurrence within 3 months [19]. A summary of risk factors for common UTIs is shown in **Table 1** [20–23].

For different reasons, postmenopausal women with the risk of developing UTIs, such as lower levels of systemic estrogen, play essential roles in adjusting the vaginal pH and maintaining the normal vaginal flora. The lower estrogen level in postmenopausal women is a crucial factor contributing to UTIs in the community. Based on a Cochrane review, vaginal estrogen, cranberries, Hyaluronic acid, and Chondroitin sulfate have a big part in decreasing recurrent UTIs [24]. Probiotics are thought to contribute to preventing UTIs by restoring the normal vaginal microbiome [25].

3. Pathogenicity and virulence factors

In the 1990s, Kloos and Bannerman [26] shed light on the clinical importance of CoNS. Today, CoNS represent one of the most virulent nosocomial pathogens which had a crucial impact on human health [27]. *Staphylococci* colonize and develop complications by owning the strain-specific virulence strategies for the aggression, invasion, and adherence factors essential for pathogenicity and evading the host immunity mechanisms. Once the periurethral region contaminated with *S. saprophyticus* from the gut, the microorganisms will colonize the urethra before traveling up to the bladder. To attach to the uroepithelial cells, *S. saprophyticus* expresses adhesins: extracellular slime and fibronectin binding proteins [27]. *S. saprophyticus strains can also produce urease which hydrolyzes the ammonia to ammonia and carbon dioxide, ammonia will support the bacteria's survival with the pH increasing* [28]. As soon as the host immune system cells sense the bacterial infection, phagocytes, macrophages and neutrophils are being called to engulf the bacteria, then the bacteria are trapped inside a phagosome, which occurs when the phagosome fuses with a specialized vesicle that has degradative agents. However, *S. saprophyticus* bacteria can eventually escape the digestion pocket in coating themselves with the hosts proteins in order to disguise themselves to prevent from being identified by antibodies or blood proteins [27].

3.1 Adherence to surface and biofilm formation

Biofilm production has a significant role in infection. It's an accumulation of microorganisms (primarily endogenous) and their self-developed polymeric matrix extracellular products which form on the surface. (e.g., the ureteral stents) The first moment of *Staphylococci* colony formation is adherence to host epithelium cells which increases its virulence and also its antibiotic tolerance in comparison with isolates without biofilm production. Adherence is critical in initiating UTI pathogenesis [28]. The colonization of the multilayered biofilm is considered an essential step in the pathogenesis of a foreign host [29]. In the biofilm, bacterial cell agglomerates, extracellular DNA (eDNA), pili, flagella, and extracellular polymeric substances are encased in an extracellular material composed of teichoic acids to protect the microorganism from the host immune system [30]. After insertion into the host, ions, polysaccharides, and other components diffuse toward the host cells and provide a receptor site for bacterial adhesins, enhancing the adherence rate. In the next step, bacterial cells release protons as signaling molecules to develop a concentration on the surface, which can lead to the formation of a biofilm format. Members of *Staphylococcus* produce various adhesins, such as proteinaceous ones, grouped into surface-anchored proteins, also termed cell wall-anchored (CWA) proteins [31].

In many developing countries the UTIs caused by *S. saprophyticus* and the structure of biofilm are not that well studied but the phases of biofilm formation by CoNS can be divided into initial attachment, Accumulation, Maturation, Detachment, and dispersal. The initial extension of CoNS is followed by the accumulation phase, which includes cell proliferation, intracellular adhesion, and maturation. A developed biofilm is built up of three layers: linking film, which cattachtch to the surface of the tissue, forming a base layer of compact microorganisms, and surface film, where free-floating bacterial cells are spread over the surface [32]. Some *Staphylococci* strains have been associated with a 240-kDa protein called biofilm-associated protein (Bap), which mediates the attachment and biofilm accumulation and plays a role in developing bacterial inflammation, recurrent cystitis, and chronic prostatitis [33]. The surface virulence factors include proteins such as Aas (Binds to the fibronectin), UafA (Binds to bladder epithelia cells), UafB (Binds to fibronectin and bladder epithelial cells), Srdl (Binds to collagen) [32]. The chosen antibiotic in uncomplicated *S. saprophyticus* UTIs is nitrofurantoin 100 mg orally twice daily for five to seven days in more complicated cases [30]. Also the prescribing of Trimethoprim-sulfamethoxazole (TMP-SMX) may be given alternatively in uncomplicated cases [30]. The general steps of biofilm formation in *S. saprophyticus* [31].

3.2 Teichoic acids

Teichoic acids are involved in the adherence of *S. saprophyticus* to host epithelium cells, which dose-dependently is promoted by the attachment of these microorganisms, which act as a bridge between fibronectin polymer material and bacteria [34]. Teichoic acids have been shown to exert binding functions for matrix molecules in Gram-positive, including *Staphylococci*. Wall teichoic acid (WTA) is linked to the peptidoglycan (PG), composed of glycerol phosphate units, substituted at the positions of glycerol with alpha-glu-cocaine, alpha-glucose, alpha-6-D-alanyl-glucose [35].

3.3 Aggressive virulence factor

Coagulase-positive staphylococci have been isolated from more than 95% of cases of toxic shock syndrome (TSS). Toxic shock syndrome toxin-1 (TSST-1) is produced in more than 92% of cases. Compared *to S. aureus*, CoNS have much lower levels of aggressiveness and mostly are not producers of super toxin antigens. The capability of CoNS to produce exfoliate toxins has been doubted since the late 1980s [36]. TSST-1-producing coagulase-negative staphylococci were also isolated from different cases, but the illness episodes were mild recurrences of TSS since they did not meet all the TSS criteria. The strains of presumed positive toxic shock syndrome toxin 1 (TSST-1) cannot produce and exert TSST-1 [37].

3.4 Production of Lantibiotics

Lantibiotics are a group of post-translationally modified peptides that contain unusual amino acids such as lanthionine residues. Commensal staphylococci produce Lantibiotics like Nisin A (act against a wide variety of bacteria, including strains of Lactococcus, Streptococcus, and Staphylococcus), Epidermin, and Mersacidin [38]. These groups of bacteriocins are classified into cationic antimicrobial peptides (CAMPs), which are classified into two types, including Type A (e.g. Nisin, Bisin, Subtilisin, and Epidermin) and Type B (e.g. Mersacidin, Duraycin, and Cinnamycin). The production plays a role in bacterial interference, creating an ecological niche for *Staphylococci* [39]. These antibiotic peptides also include methyl xanthine amino acids, which can bind to bacterial cell wall precursor lipid components and disrupt cell wall production. Type A kills rapidly by pore-forming mechanisms, and Type B inhibits peptidoglycan biosynthesis [40].

4. Identification and grouping of CoNS by novobiocin testing

Novobiocin is an antibiotic that interferes with DNA replication and binds to DNA gyrase, leading to the blocking of adenosine triphosphates (ATPase) activity. If a CoNS isolate is recovered from urinary tract specimens, testing for resistance to novobiocin will distinguish *S. saprophyticus* from other clinical CoNS [41]. This method is based on the disc diffusion test using 5-μg novobiocin discs on Hinton agar or blood agar medium [41]. As the microorganism multiplies during incubation to produce a surface of confluent growth, cells are exposed to the antibiotic that diffuses into the agar from the paper disk. If the bacteria are susceptible to novobiocin, there will be a formation of a zone of inhibition around the disk representing an area where the bacterial growth has been prevented [42]. A zone of inhibition less than 16 mm is indicative of novobiocin resistance. The CoNS have been classified into two groups based on this particular pattern. The ones demonstrating novobiocin susceptibility include *epidermidis, S. capitis, S. haemolyticus, S. hominis, S. lugdunensis, S. warneri* and *S. saccharolyticus.* The novobiocin-resistant group consists of: *S. kloosii, S. saprophyticus,* and *S. xylosus* [42].

5. Antimicrobial susceptibility

UTIs are individually becoming challenging to treat due to the incorrectly widespread antibiotic use and bacterial resistance mechanism. Regarding antimicrobial resistance, CoNS have been divided into two groups: 1-Susceptible to antimicrobial agents and 2-those exposed to antibiotics in the hospital. CoNS are thought to show an exquisite reservoir of genetic elements that led to resistance to β-lactam antibiotics and other antimicrobial classes [43]. In *Staphylococci*, including CoNS species, penicillin-binding protein (PBP) expression can lead to β-lactam resistance, such as cephalosporins and carbapenem [44].

6. Preventing recurrent UTI/probiotics

Nonantimicrobial and antimicrobial prophylaxis regimens have been studied in the female population with recurrent UTIs. Probiotics can prevent UTIs by helping to restore the normal vaginal microbiome. Studies investing in *Lactobacillus* spp. to prevent recurrent UTIs in women have found a link between recurrent symptomatic UTIs and probiotics. Still, additional studies are needed for final decisions to be made [45].

6.1 Preventing recurrent UTI/cranberries

The mechanism of cranberries preventing UTI is yet to be discovered. Although, studies show that the daily drinking of 300 mL of cranberry juice plays a role in preventing this complication due to the function of proanthocyanidins found in cranberry, which inhibit the microorganisms from adhering to the bladder walls and the epithelium cells and make tissues damages [46].

6.2 Preventing recurrent UTI/hyaluronic acid and chondroitin sulfate

The glycosaminoglycan layer has been found in the bladder wall, made of Hyaluronic acid and Chondroitin sulfate, which plays a role in preventing the adherence of microorganisms to the urothelial cells [47]. A damaged glycosaminoglycan layer could lead to an increased rate of recurrent UTIs in both the male and female populations (**Table 2**) [48].

7. Treatment and resistance

Treatment with antibiotics has been indicated in complicated UTIs and pyelonephritis. There is no indication for routine susceptibility tests for UTI due to *S. saprophyticus* because it's usually susceptible to empirical therapy for uncomplicated UTI [49]. The antibiotics for uncomplicated UTI are sulfonamides, ampicillin, and nitrofurantoin 100 mg twice daily for five days or trimethoprim/sulfamethoxazole

Medication	Dose
Vaginal estrogen	Estradiol ring 2 mg
Probiotics	Vaginal suppositories two times a week
Cranberries	300 mL juice
Hyaluronic acid and Chondroitin sulfate	800 mg and 1 g in 50-mL solution
Antibiotics	Nitrofurantoin 50 mg daily
	TMP-SMX daily
	Cephalexin 125 mg daily
	Norfloxacin 200 mg daily

Table 2.
Prophylaxis for recurrent UTI.

160/800 twice daily for three days. In acute uncomplicated UTIs, NSAIDs are a preferred analgesic [50, 51]. resistance to trimethoprim/sulfamethoxazole can lead to failure in empirical therapy, so an antimicrobial susceptibility test is necessary in these cases [52]. Baicalin can be used in UTI treatment because of its inhibitory effects on more efflux gene expression, which encode the msrA efflux pump, which is essential in multidrug resistance in staphylococcus strains [52]. Nalidixic acid has no rule in treating *S. saprophyticus* UTI due to bacterial resistance. In some studies, the terms methicillin resistance and Oxacillin resistance is being used and recording to CLSI guideline the cefoxitin disc is also being used [54]. Oxacillin resistance occurs due to the production of pB2a in the microbe [52]. Pivmecillinam is another acceptable antibiotic in pregnant patients, while mecillinam is not practical [54] (**Table 3**).

A single dose of fosfomycin trometamol also is a good choice in treating uncomplicated UTI and pregnant patients with lower UTI as a first-line empirical therapy (**Figure 2**) [53].

Some *S. saprophyticus* species are resistant to Cefixime and fosfomycin trometamol naturally, so it does not recommend to use these drugs in treating acute

Antibiotic	Dose
Nitrofurantoin monohydrate	100 mg
TMP-SMX	160/800 mg
Fosfomycin	3 g once
Pivmecillinam	400 mg
Fluoroquinolones	Ciprofloxacin 250 mg
	Ofloxacin 200 mg
Amoxicillin-clavulanate	500/125 mg
Cephalosporins	Cefdinir 100 mg
	Cefaclor 250 mg
	Cefpodoxime
Ciprofloxacin	500 mg

Table 3.
Treatment with antibiotics.

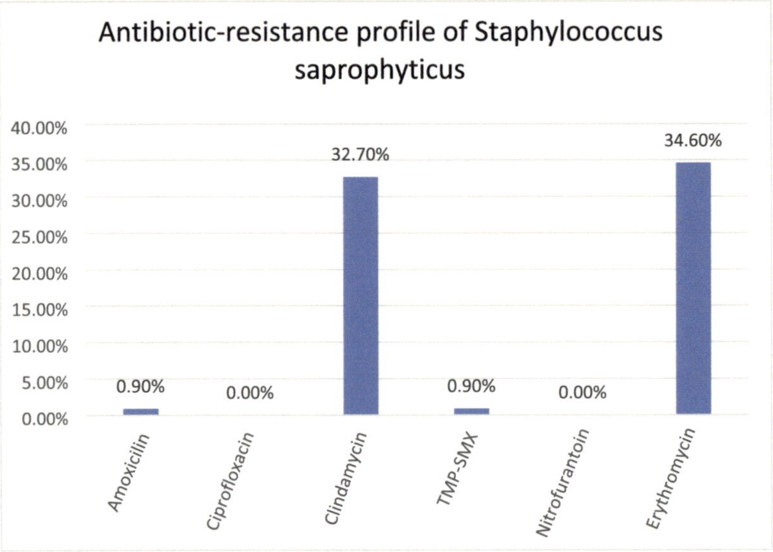

Figure 2.
Antibiotic-resistance profile [54].

pyelonephritis. Ceftriaxone can be used instead of Cefixime and ciprofloxacin for treating acute pyelonephritis [55].

8. Conclusion

CoNS are versatile Gram-positive bacteria, either coagulase-positive or coagulase-negative, with mucous membranes and skin niches. Coagulase-negative organisms should not always be thought of as contaminants in tissue infection. CoNS rarely get hostile because most of them lack virulence factors. Based on the rise of weak and susceptible patients, CoNS consequently have become major nosocomial pathogens, and their virulence functions have led to complications such as urinary tract infections (UTI). Urinary tract infections are among the most frequent types of hospital and community infections especially in women than man because of their anatomical differences. Pyelonephritis and cystitis are the most common UTIs based on the factors affecting patients and are classified as complicated or uncomplicated. Uncomplicated infections are those in nonpregnant healthy women with normal genitourinary tract and medical history without any recent UTIs. *S. saprophyticus* is one of the major pathogens causing UTIs. It is a Coagulase-negative Staphylococci (CoNS), colonizing the ureter epithelium via adhesins with the ability to produce biofilms to increase their pathogenicity, however little has being discovered about antibiotic resistant patterns and biofilm functions in this topic. We must know that the treatment of UTIs depends on the S. saprophyticus growing resistance to antibiotics. The big part of *S. saprophyticus* infections can be treated with antibiotics as said before but if left untreated, can progress to complications. A great deal of knowledge of antimicrobial resistance patterns is essential when choosing an antibiotic agent. So many questions about the ecology, pathogenesis, and phylogeny of CoNS have not been answered yet, but hopefully, following the development of new methodology tools, further research can be approached.

Author details

Benyamin Djawadi[1*], Nazila Heidari[2] and Mojtaba Mohseni[3]

1 Faculty of Medical Sciences, Parasitology Department, Tarbiat Modares University, Iran

2 Department of Medical Science, Iran University of Medical Sciences, Tehran, Iran

3 Department of Microbiology, University of Mazandaran, Babolsar, Iran

*Address all correspondence to: benyamin_djawadi@modares.ac.ir

References

[1] Argemi X, Hansmann Y, Prola K, Prevost G. Coagulase-negative *Staphylococci pathogenomics*. International Journal of Molecular Sciences. 11 Mar 2019;**20**(5):1215

[2] Pinault L, Chabrière E, Raoult D, Fenollar F. Direct identification of pathogens in urine by use of a specific matrix-assisted laser desorption ionization–Time of flight spectrum database. Journal of Clinical Microbiology. 28 Mar 2019;57(4):e01678-18

[3] Natsis N, Cohen P. Coagulase-negative *Staphylococcus* skin and soft tissue infections. American Journal of Clinical Dermatology. Oct 2018;**19**(5):671-677

[4] Lala V, Leslie S, Minter D. Acute Cystitis. MSU-McLaren Oakland: StatPearls; 2022

[5] Hur J, Lee A, Hong J, Cho O-H. *Staphylococcus saprophyticus* bacteremia originating from urinary tract infections: A case report and literature review. Infect Chemother. Jun 2016;**48**(2):136-139

[6] Mireles A, Walker J, Caparon M, Hultgren S. Urinary tract infections: Epidemiology, mechanisms of infection and treatment options. Nature Reviews Microbiology. May 2015;**13**(5):269-284

[7] Nicolle L. A practical guide to the management of complicated urinary. Drugs. Apr 1997;**53**(4):583-592

[8] Foxman B, Barlow R. Urinary tract infection: Selfreported incidence and associated costs. Annals of Epidemiology. Nov 2000;**10**(8):509-515

[9] Hooton T, Stapleton A. A prospective study of asymptomatic bacteriuria in young sexually active women. The New England Journal of Medicine. 5 Oct 2000;**343**(14):992-997

[10] Sobel J. Pathogenesis of urinary tract infection: Role of host defenses. Infectious Disease Clinics of North America. Sep 1997;**11**(3):531-549

[11] Patterson J, Andriole V. Bacterial urinary tract infections in diabetes. Infectious Disease Clinics of North America. Sep 1997;**11**(3):735-750

[12] Stamm W. Prevention of urinary tract infection. Infectious Disease Clinics of North America. Sep 1997;**11**(3):719-733

[13] Bonkat G, Pickard B, Bartoletti R. European association of urology guidelines on urological infections. 2018. [Online]. Available from: http://uroweb.org/guideline/urological-infections. [Accessed 7 August 2018]

[14] Hooton T. Uncomplicated urinary tract infection. The New England Journal of Medicine. 15 Mar 2012;**366**(11):1028-1037

[15] Gupta K, Hooton T, Naber K, Colgan R, Miller L, Moran G, et al. International clinical practice guidelines for the treatment of acute uncomplicated cystitis and pyelonephritis in women: A 2010 update by the infectious diseases society of America and the European society for microbiology and infectious diseases. Clinical Infectious Disease. 2011;**52**(5):103-120

[16] Knottnerus B, Geerlings S. Women with symptoms of uncomplicated urinary tract infection are often willing to delay antibiotic treatment. BMC Family Practice. 31 May 2013;**14**:71

[17] Solomon C. Acute pyelonephritis in adults. The New England Journal of Medicine. 2018:48-59

[18] Albert X, Huertas E, Pereiro I, Sanfélix J. Antibiotics for preventing recurrent urinary tract infection in non-pregnant women. The Cochrane Database of Systematic Reviews. 2004;(3)

[19] Dason S, Dason JT, Kapoor A. A Guidelines for the diagnosis and management of recurrent urinary tract infection in women. Canadian Urological Association Journal. Oct 2011;**5**(5):316-322

[20] Juthani-Mehta M. Urinary tract infections in older women: A clinical review. JAMA. Feb 2014:844-854

[21] Raz R, Gennesin Y, Wasser J. Recurrent urinary tract infections in postmenopausal women. Clinical Infectious Diseases. 2000:152-156

[22] Perrotta C, Mejia R. Oestrogens for preventing recurrent urinary tract infection in postmenopausal women. Cochrane Database of Systematic Reviews. 16 Apr 2008;(2):CD005131

[23] Nallamothu B, Fihn S. Does this woman have an acute uncomplicated urinary tract infection? JAMA. 2002;**287**(20):2701-2710

[24] Devillé W, Yzermans J. The urine dipstick test useful to rule out infections. A meta-analysis of the accuracy. BMC Urology. 2 Jun 2004;**4**:4

[25] Schwenger E. Probiotics for preventing urinary tract infections in adults and children. Cochrane Database of Systematic Reviews. 23 Dec 2015;**2015**(12)

[26] Kloos W, Bannerman T. Update on clinical significance of coagulase-negative staphylococci. Clinical Microbiology Reviews. Jan 1994;7(1):117-140

[27] Garduño E, Blanco J, Said I, Beteta A, Márquez I. *Staphylococcus saprophyticus* causing native valve endocarditis. Scandinavian Journal of Infectious Diseases. 2005;**37**(9):690-691

[28] Peters G, Pulverer G. Adherence and growth of coagulase-negative *Staphylococci* on surfaces of intravenous catheters. The Journal of Infectious Diseases. Oct 1982;**146**(4):479-482

[29] Christensen G, Simpson A. Adherence of slime-producing strains of *Staphylococcus* epidermidis to smooth surfaces. Infection and Immunity. Jul 1982;**37**(1):318-326

[30] Izano E, Amarante M, Kher W, Keplan J. Differential roles of poly-N-acetylglucosamine surface polysaccharide and extracellular DNA in Staphylococcus aureus and *Staphylococcus* epidermidis biofilms. Applied and Environmental Microbiology. Jan 2008;**74**(2):470-476

[31] Heilmann C. Adhesion mechanisms of *Staphylococci*. Advances in Experimental Medicine and Biology. 2011;**715**:105-123

[32] Greenberg P, Stewart P. Bacterial biofilms: A common cause of persistent infections. Science. 1999

[33] Cucaralla C, Solano C, Valle J, Amorena B. Bap, a *Staphylococcus aureus* surface protein involved in biofilm formation. Journal of Bacteriology. May 2001;**183**(9):2888-2896

[34] Herrmann M, Herrmann C. Teichoic acid enhances adhesion of *Staphylococcus epidermidis* to immobilized fibronectin. Microbial Pathogenesis. Dec 2001;**31**(6):261-270

[35] Sadovskaya I, Jabbouri S, Li J, Vinogradov E. Structural elucidation of the extracellular and cell-wall teichoic

acids of *Staphylococcus epidermidis* RP62A, a reference biofilm-positive strain. Carbohydrate Research. 1 Jun 2004;**339**(8):1467-1473

[36] Kahler R, Boyce J. Toxic shock syndrome associated with TSST-1 producing coagulase-negative *staphylococci*. The American Journal of the Medical Sciences. Nov 1986;**292**(5):310-312

[37] Villani F, Casaburi A. PCR detection of staphylococcal enterotoxin genes in *Staphylococcus* spp. strains isolated from meat and dairy products. Evidence for new variants of seG and seI in *S. aureus* AB-8802. Journal of Applied Microbiology. 2004;**97**(4):719-730

[38] Götz F, Schlag M, Werne R, Popella P, Perconti S. Epidermin and gallidermin: *Staphylococcal lantibiotics*. International Journal of Medical Microbiology. Jan 2014;**304**(1):63-71

[39] Bierbaum G. Lantibiotics: Biosynthesis and biological activities of uniquely modified peptides from gram-positive bacteria. Annual Review of Microbiology. 1998;**52**:41-79

[40] Götz F, Schlag M. *Staphylococcal lantibiotics*. International Journal of Medical Microbiology. Jan 2014;**304**(1):63-71

[41] Thornsberry C, Hébert A. Characteristics of coagulase-negative staphylococci that help differentiate these species and other members of the family Micrococcaceae. Journal of Clinical Microbiology. Oct 1988;**26**(10):1939-1949

[42] Becker K. Manual of Clinical Microbiology 12th edition. Vol. 12011

[43] CLSI. Performance standards for antimicrobial susceptibility testing; 23rd Informational Supplement. The Clinical and Laboratory Standards Institute. 2013

[44] Tomasz A, Hartman B. Low-affinity penicillin-binding protein associated with beta-lactam resistance. Journal of Bacteriology. 1984

[45] Kolman K. Cystitis and Pyelonephritis: Diagnosis, Treatment, and Prevention, Prime Care. 2019

[46] Jepson R, Williams G. Cranberries for preventing urinary tract infections. Cochrane, 2012. [Online]. Available from: Cochranelibrary.com

[47] Damiano R, Autorino R, Domenico R, Quarto G, Bava I, Ucciero G. Prevention of recurrent urinary tract infections by intravesical administration of hyaluronic acid and chondroitin sulphate: A placebo-controlled randomised trial. European Urology. 2011;**59**(4):645-651

[48] Vita D, Giordano S. Effectiveness of intravesical hyaluronic acid/chondroitin sulfate in recurrent bacterial cystitis: A randomized study. International Urogynecology Journal. Dec 2012;**23**(12):1707-1713

[49] Ferreira A, Cunha M, Camargo C, Mondelli A, Bonesso M. Oxacillin resistance and antimicrobial susceptibility profile of *Staphylococcus saprophyticus* and other *staphylococci* isolated from patients with urinary tract infection. Chemotherapy. 2012;**58**(6):482-491

[50] Hooton T, Dilanchian P. Diagnosis, treatment, and prevention of urinary tract infection. Microbiology Spectrum. Dec 2016;**4**(6)

[51] Mårdh A, Hovelius B. *Staphylococcus saprophyticus* as a common cause of urinary tract infections. 1984;**6**(3):328-337

[52] Wang J, Jiao H, Meng J, Qiao M, Wang D, Du H, et al. Baicalin inhibits biofilm formation and the

quorum-sensing system by regulating the MsrA drug efflux pump in *Staphylococcus saprophyticus*. Frontiers in Microbiology. 10 Dec 2019;**10**:2800

[53] Pailhoriès H, Lemarié C, Eveillard M, Kempf M, Chenouard R, Cassisa V. *Staphylococcus saprophyticus*: Which beta-lactam? International Journal of Infectious Diseases. Dec 2017;**65**:63-66

[54] Adeghate J, Juhasz E, Pongracz J, Rimanoczy E, Kristof K. Does *Staphylococcus saprophyticus* cause acute cystitis only in young females, or is there more to the story? A one-year comprehensive study done in budapest, hungary. Acta Microbiologica et Immunologica Hungarica. Mar 2016;**63**(1):57-67

[55] Keating G. Fosfomycin trometamol: A review of its use as a single-dose oral treatment for patients with acute lower urinary tract infections and pregnant women with asymptomatic bacteriuria. Drugs. Nov 2013;**73**(17):1951-1966

Chapter 3

Urinary Tract Infection in HIV/AIDS Patients

Gerardo Amaya-Tapia, Gabriela Ibarra-Nieto, Octavio Campollo Rivas and José Luis González Sánchez

Abstract

Urinary tract infection (UTI) is a common condition around the world, even affecting immunocompromised hosts such as people with human immunodeficiency virus (HIV) infection or acquired immuodeficiency syndrome (AIDS). Due to the anatomical conditions of the urogenital tract, women are more susceptible to UTI. Risk factors throughout life are determinants in the appearance of UTI. The frequency increases especially in women and is associated with sexual activity and pregnancy. In older adults and the elderly, again the frequency of UTI in both genders increases. In women, it is usually related at anatomical and functional sequelae due to parity and gyneco-obstetric surgeries. In old men, prostatic enlargement is an important concern. Chronic degenerative diseases such as diabetes mellitus with complications explain the high frequency of UTI in this population. Currently, the increase in violence and accidents are the leading cause of traumatic injuries with neurological damage, which leads the use of permanent urinary catheter. In patients infected with HIV/AIDS, the disease can be severe and is associated with more complications. The etiology in this population can be diverse, including fungi, parasites, and virus; antimicrobial resistance is a therapeutic challenge. This chapter is a comprehensive review of the epidemiology, pathophysiology, clinical presentation, diagnosis approach, and current treatment of UTIs in HIV/AIDS patients.

Keywords: urinary tract infection, UTIs, HIV, AIDS, HIV/AIDS

1. Introduction

UTI is defined as the presence of some pathogenic microorganism that induces a local or systemic inflammatory response. The infection can affect any structure of the urinary tract including the renal parenchyma, pelvic, ureters, bladder, and urethra. In general, infections located above the ureterovesical junction are considered as high infections and below this junction are considered as low. High-location UTIs are considered more severe but less frequent, and their exact location is often difficult to determine. UTI is considered the most common bacterial infection, estimated to affect more than 150 million people annually [1]. From 15 to 50 years of age, UTI is practically nonexistent in men, while in women, it has a prevalence that can reach up to 3% of the population [2]. Approximately, one in three women suffers an uncomplicated UTI before the age of 24 years old, and 30–44% develop a recurrent disease [3].

IntechOpen

People living with HIV are more likely to develop UTIs due to the suppression of their immunity. AIDS is considered the late stage of HIV infection, when the number of the CD4 cells falls below 200 cells/mm^3 or when patients develop one or more opportunistic infections regardless of their low CD4 count. The incidence of UTI is increased in HIV patients, but there is a significant variance in the reported prevalence. Evidence suggests that HIV infection is associated with UTIs and abnormalities of bladder function, which is demonstrated by urodynamic studies [4, 5]. However, it is unclear whether HIV/AIDS imposes an additional risk of urinary conditions beyond the normal risk associated with age or other risk factors.

The urinary tract may be susceptible to complications of HIV infection [6], with *Escherichia coli* and *Enterobacter* spp. being found to be the dominant pathogens associated with UTIs [7]. Unusual germs such as *Salmonella* and *Acinetobacter* have also been reported. Other atypical pathogens such as fungi, *Toxoplasma gondii*, mycobacteria, cytomegalovirus (CMV), and adenovirus are often disseminated at the time of urinary tract infection, usually when CD4 counts are $<100/mm^3$ [8–10].

Opportunistic infections are well described in patients with HIV infection, but infections that do not define AIDS are relatively understudied. The diversity of microorganisms that can cause UTIs and the magnitude of drug resistance may cause treatment choices to be significantly limited. Improving knowledge on the prevalence, uropathogen spectrum, and associated factors of UTIs could substantially improve the current diagnostic and treatment guidelines for better prognosis of people living with HIV/AIDS.

2. Epidemiology

UTI is a disease of high prevalence worldwide, accounting for 150 million infections per year [11], and UTI hospital-acquired infections account for 40% of all hospital infections worldwide [12]. Indwelling urinary catheterization is the most common risk factor for hospital-complicated UTI [13].

Age and gender are conditions that impact the frequency of UTIs prominently. Risk factors are variable at certain stages of life; women suffer from UTIs more often than men, with nearly half of women developing UTIs throughout their lives [14]. Anatomical and physiological differences, such as a shorter urethra and hormone fluctuations, explain the high frequency of UTIs in women [15]. This pronounced increase in susceptibility in women is more remarkable in adolescents, pregnant women, and adults under 50 years of age. In populations older than 65 years, the prevalence of bacteriuria and UTI increases substantially in men to almost equal that of elderly women [16, 17].

HIV/AIDS continues to be a major problem throughout the world. New infections continue to occur in a significant way in conjunction with other sexually transmitted diseases (STIs) such as syphilis, papillomavirus, viral hepatitis, and many others. The ignored pandemic, alcoholism, drug addiction, sexual promiscuity, and violence has caused the increase and appearance of many diseases, including the emerging monkeypox infection and other diseases previously mentioned. This scenario has brought fatal consequences on the health and economy of many countries. Poverty and mental health issues (depression) are an important part of this vicious circle.

According to World Health Organization (WHO) data, there were an estimated 38.4 million (33.9–43.8 million) people living with HIV at the end 2021, two-thirds of whom were in the African region. In 2021, 650,000 people died of HIV-related causes, and 1.5 million (1.1–2.0 million) people acquired HIV. In our current time frame, it is estimated that 40.1 million people have died from HIV-related causes [18]. There are many reports on the prevalence of UTI in HIV/AIDS-infected patients, some with a small number of patients and with limitations in the design of their studies. Most of the information comes from observational studies conducted over some period or cross-sectionally. As patients' ages are diverse, it is difficult to separate the inherent risk associated with their age and gender. Most studies do not include a control group (people who do not have HIV infection) to determine the risk.

The most cited research is the article published by Miles and associates [19], where they refer to an incidence of 17% of UTIs; however, the article was published in 1989. Due to the little information and the absence of well-designed studies to establish this knowledge, Miles' article is still taken as the main reference. The article was done retrospectively in a hospital in Detroit, Michigan, USA, with 120 patients seen from 1984 to 1987, practically at the beginning of the HIV pandemic. Only 16% of the patients had some urinary symptom, and at least one urine culture was performed in 56 of 120 patients, in which 17 (14%) were positive.

There is a consensus that people with lower CD4 have a high risk of developing UTIs as well as other opportunistic infections. The female sex constitutes an additional risk to the immunological state. The number of partners and sexual orientation are surely additional factors of risk of UTIs; however, there are no publications that provide sufficient clarity in this regard.

In patients with HIV who are hospitalized for any cause, the prevalence of hospital-acquired UTI increases significantly. In a study with 96 patients, of which 78 (81%) were men who were divided by the diagnosis of AIDS or HIV infection, the prevalence in patients with AIDS was 50% and in patients with HIV infection was 13.6%. From 18 women, 67% suffered from UTIs versus 35% of men ($p = 0.03$). The study included a control group without HIV in which the prevalence of UTI was 11.7% [7]. Studies on UTI prevalence in HIV/AIDS patients are shown in **Table 1**.

Author (year)	Ref	Patient number	Age range (y)	CD4 < 200 (%)	CV <10^5 log (%)	UTI number (%)
Miles (1989)	[19]	120	N.A.	N.A.	N.A.	17 (14)
Schönwald S. (1999)	[7]	96 (74 AIDS, 22 HIV)	16–68 (100%)	N.A.	N.A	(50) AIDS (13.6) HIV
Omoregie R. (2009)	[20]	421 (317 HIV vs. 104 non HIV)	N.A.	30	N.A.	(27) HIV (13) non HIV
De Pinho A. (1994)	[21]	415 (151 AIDS, 94 HIV, 170 non HIV)	18–50 (100%)	N.A,	N.A.	10 (6.6) in AIDS, none in both HIV and non HIV
Yepes A. (2010)	[22]	237	20–50 (70%)	61.5	76.9	13 (5.4)
Boaitey Y. (2012)	[23]	800 (500 HIV vs. 300 non HIV)	20–50 (61%)	N.A.	N.A.	5 (1) in HIV and 2 (0.7) in non HIV
Mota L. (2022)	[24]	57	20–30 (70%)	N.A	N.A.	30 (53)

N.A. = not available.

Table 1.
Prevalence of UTI in HIV/AIDS patients.

In a recent systematic review and meta-analysis about the magnitude and associated factors of UTIs among adults living with HIV in Ethiopia, seven studies were selected with 2257 participants that met the selection criteria. All were observational studies with an overall prevalence of 12.8% (range 10.3–18% for all studies). Additionally, it analyzed some risk factors such as gender, diabetes mellitus, history of catheterization, and CD4 counts. Those with CD4 counts larger than 200 had a lower risk of UTI than those with CD4 counts less than 200 (OR: 0.36, 95% CI: 0.06–2.35) with statistical significance of P = 0.001 [25].

3. Pathogenesis

Urinary tract infections usually migrate through the urethra, and microorganisms colonize the periurethral region. In a simple case, microorganisms can arrive in the urinary tract through the blood in the presence of a systemic disease such as perinephric abscess, renal tuberculosis, and some mycoses. A UTI may involve any site of the urinary tract, including renal parenchyma, renal pelvis, ureters, bladder, and urethra. Infection of the renal parenchyma is termed pyelonephritis. The infection of the upper urinary tract is usually associated with severe disease.

The ascent of bacteria colonizing the urethral meatus is more common in women due to the short urethra and bacterial colonization in adjacent vulvar and perianal regions [26]. Sometimes, a specific risk factor is present, such as pregnancy, indwelling catheter drainage or intermittent urinary catheterization of the bladder due to paraplegia, neurogenic bladder, bladder outlet obstruction, prostatism, urethral stricture, analgesic abuse neuropathy, or ureteral stricture from recurrent renal colic. Some of this risk factors can be inferred from proper questioning [27, 28]. The human body is host to a wide variety of microorganisms, establishing a well-known symbiotic relation [29]. Extensive studies on human microbiome have generated an unprecedented understanding of the microorganisms that colonize both the human body and its external environment [30].

Uropathogenic reservoirs often prevail within the urinary tract and the surrounding vaginal and gut microbiomes, causing recurrent UTIs in up to 30% of individuals within 6 months of the initial infection [31]. Urotypes in the female urobiome are commonly dominated by *Shigella*, *Lactobacillus*, *Enterococcus*, *Gardnerella*, *Prevotella*, and *E. coli*. The paradigm that has existed for years stating that urine is a liquid sterile under normal conditions has now been refuted by recent studies in which flora has been found in the bladder of adult woman [32, 33].

Specific virulence factors and various pathogens that cause UTIs have been studied extensively [34, 35]. Certain strains of *E. coli*, called uropathogenics, have been implicated as the most prevalent bacterium causing ITUs in different populations. *E. coli* adherence to uroepithelium is mediated by adhesins such as pili or fimbriae, interacting with specific receptors expressed on the surface of the uroepithelial cells. Fimbriated strains of *E. coli* account for 90% of pyelonephritis, and is the most predominant strain of bacteremic cases. Cell wall O antigens, capsular polysaccharide K antigens, and the flagellar H antigens have been associated with UTI severity. Other bacterial virulence factors associated with UTIs include aerobactin, hemolysins, and cytotoxic necrotizing factors [34, 35].

However, a high rate of UTIs has been described in patients with advanced HIV [7, 21]. Bacteriuria with the consequent risk of UTI has been found in >30% in patients living with HIV who have CD4 < 200 cell/mm^3 [36]. A routine study in this population is recommended specially in advanced disease. Urine cultures may be negative because the patient is taking prophylactic antimicrobials against opportunistic infections. Urine should be cultured for mycobacteria, and the use of special culture media and stains, blood cultures, and viral titers should be considered [9, 37]. Intravenous pyelogram, renal ultrasound, or abdominal computed tomography may be very useful, and tissue biopsies may be necessary to establish a diagnosis, for example, CMV cystitis [8, 38].

Immune status is decisive in the occurrence of opportunistic infections; the critical levels associated with the occurrence of opportunistic infections are below 200 CD4/mm^3 cells in the blood. Following initial infection, HIV spreads to regional lymph nodes within 3–6 days due to the large population of HIV-targeted CD4+ T cells and constant cell trafficking by lymphatic vessels; systemic dissemination occurs, and studies suggest that the lymph node reservoir may be established within the first 2 weeks of infection (6–25 days) [39–41]. Viral replication is associated with a decline in the CD4 cell count and immune system deterioration. High viral load and low CD4 cell count are associated with a greater risk of opportunistic infections and progression to AIDS. HIV has been isolated from blood and many other fluids and secretions [37].

Therapeutic interventions that decrease plasma HIV RNA levels are associated with an improved prognosis [42, 43]. Since the first antiretroviral (ARV) was produced three decades ago, ARV therapy has transformed HIV infection from inevitable immune collapse and death into a chronic disease that can now be treated and prevented with a pill taken once a day [44]. Despite these advances, the definitive cure is still pending [45, 46].

4. Clinic presentation and risk factors

The clinical presentation of UTIs in patients with HIV/AIDS infection does not appear to be different from that described in the general population; the infection would be expected to be more severe in immunosuppressed patients, and signs and symptoms of UTI may be mild because there is no inflammatory response to infection. The specific clinical manifestations may be more related to the etiology and location of the UTI where variations in the clinical presentation are to be expected. The health consequences of UTI among HIV-infected patients can be severe, resulting in acute and chronic kidney diseases [47], infertility, cancer, sepsis, and neurologic complication, which lead to urinary stasis [48].

Fever, dysuria, and polyuria are the most frequent symptoms of UTIs; the presence of any of these symptoms is indicative of a UTI in about 50% of cases. The combination of symptoms increases the probability of a UTI to over 90% [49]. Low-location UTIs such as cystitis are the most frequent, least aggressive, and least related to factors that are predisposed to recurrences. On the other hand, high-location UTIs (such as pyelonephritis) are usually less frequent but more aggressive and can include sudden onset with bacteremia and high fever and may be present with signs and symptoms such as costovertebral pain and macroscopic hematuria [19, 50]. Both cystitis and pyelonephritis are complicated when they occur in the presence of a condition that increases the risk of recurrence or when are caused by resistant pathogens.

Cystitis can be defined as an infection of the urinary bladder accompanied by symptoms of dysuria, frequency, and urgency. Chronic pyelonephritis is commonly found in association with other renal diseases, such as chronic obstruction, uric acid nephropathy, analgesic abuse, and hypokalemic nephropathy. Acute bacterial prostatitis generally presents with abrupt onset of fever, chills, dysuria, frequency, urgency, as well as perineal pain with symptoms of irritative and obstructive voiding dysfunction. Relapsing episodes of UTIs, either cystitis or pyelonephritis, are common [51].

Urosepsis may be defined as symptomatic bacteremia of urinary tract origin. It is a rare but life-threatening complication of UTI. Community-acquired urosepsis in an otherwise healthy host typically arises from acute pyelonephritis or renal abscess [52]. Hemorrhagic cystitis is characterized by hematuria, dysuria, frequency, and urgency, and in severe cases, blood clots can result in bladder outlet obstruction. This condition is generally associated with BK virus, adenovirus infection in bone marrow, and kidney transplant recipients, and it occurs in the early transplant period [53–55].

Clinical manifestations, etiology, and recurrence can also change widely in relation to host conditions, such as pregnancy, malformations of the urinary tract, and presence of lithiasis or tumor. Aging affects the function of all organs and systems and the urinary tract is not an exception. Prostate growth, neurogenic bladder with urinary retention, and increase frequency of asymptomatic bacteriuria are common at this stage of life [52]. An important part of the population living with HIV are people over 65 years of age who, like the rest of the population, suffer from chronic degenerative diseases.

In a previous cohort [56] of 33,336 male veterans with UTI, 234 (0.7%) were diagnosed with HIV infection. Patients with HIV were significantly younger than those without HIV (56.5 vs. 68.0 years; $P < .001$). Among the assessed comorbidities known or hypothesized to be associated with UTI, several differences between patients with HIV versus patients without HIV were observed (**Table 2**). Although this study represents a very specific population, it allows to consider the most common comorbidities that can be associated with UTIs in men who are non-HIV-infected compared with those who are HIV-infected.

Catheter-associated urinary tract infection (CAUTI) is defined as the new appearance of bacteriuria or funguria at a concentration greater than 10^5 CFU mL

Comorbidity	**NonHIV (33,102)**	**HIV infected (n = 234)**	***P* value**
Diabetes mellitus	34.7	23.1	<.001
Benign prostatic hypertrophy	33.1	19.2	<.001
Prior UTI	30.9	27.3	.25
Incontinence	16.3	13.2	.20
Chronic kidney disease	10.8	11.5	.72
Prostate cancer	11.1	7.7	.10
Urethral stricture	7.8	4.3	.047
Urinary calculi	7.0	9.0	.24
Spinal cord injury	4.0	3.4	.32
Prostatitis	2.6	5.1	.02
Vesicoureteral reflux	0.1	0	.63

Adapted from: Drekonja et al. [56].

Table 2.
Percent of comorbidities associated with UTIs among non-HIV and HIV infected male patients.

according to the Centers for Disease Control and Prevention. More than 75% of hospital-acquired or nosocomial urinary tract infections are initiated by urinary catheters, which are used during the treatment of 15–25% of hospitalized patients. Infection occurs in 10–50% of patients undergoing non-Foley or short-term urinary catheterization (7 days), but virtually all patients undergoing Foley or long-term catheterization (>28 days) become infected [57]. There are different risk factors for CAUTI; one of the main reason for this condition is the material used in the fabrication of urinary catheters that allows colonization by microorganisms and subsequent bacteriuria and infection, especially for long-term catheterization [58]. Although there is a large amount of research on CAUTI, the ideal catheter with biocompatible, antimicrobial, and antifouling materials has not yet been developed [58].

The clinical manifestations of a patient with CAUTI may pass unnoticed or be present in a severe way. Evidence suggests that the diagnosis of CAUTI based on clinical signs varies widely among clinicians and is often inaccurate when compared to published guidelines [59, 60]. Clinical practice guidelines identify several such indicators, including fever, suprapubic tenderness, flank tenderness, and delirium [13]. Unfortunately, standardized procedures to assess some of these indicators have not yet been described in the literature, and information about the consistency of some of these assessment findings from one clinician to another is yet to be reported [61]. In a study of CAUTI assessment profile, three clinical manifestations, fever, suprapubic tenderness, and delirium, had acceptable and statistically significant consistency between three nurse rates, while flank tenderness did not [62].

Infection is a common precipitating factor for delirium, particularly in the elderly [63, 64]. Delirium is defined as an acute change in cognitive status resulting from an underlying medical, psychiatric, environmental, or multifactorial cause. This manifestation of CAUTI has four indicators: acute onset with a fluctuating course, inattention, disorganized thinking, and altered level of consciousness. In a study of 210 admissions, 72 (15%) HIV-infected patients had higher rates of infection compared with their overall nosocomial rates of 6.9%. This study showed that the use of urinary catheters, gastrointestinal procedures, and vascular access were the risk factors for hospital-acquired infection [65].

In a prospective cohort between February 1998 and October 1999 in a Brazilian infectious disease unit, 257 HIV-infected patients were matched with a control group of 204 HIV-negative patients by age, diagnosis, severity of illness, and prior hospitalization. The rates of hospital acquired infections (HAI) in the studied group were 8.16 for HIV-positive patients and 3.94 for HIV-negative patients per 1000 patient days ($P = .01$). Bloodstream infections, UTIs, vascular infections, and pneumonia were the most common diseases. Three UTIs were detected in HIV-positive patients and 7 in HIV-negative patients. Although HIV-positive patients were more likely to use a urinary tract catheter, there was no difference between both groups regarding the incidence of UTIs. No clinical picture and CD4 data were provided [66]. The education of competent healthcare workers is essential in CAUTI prevention. Its effectiveness is shown especially in comprehensive and contain information course about correct procedures of urinary bladder catheterization [67]. A well-working team of HAI prevention experts in hospitals with high-quality and comprehensively provided nursing care is essential [68].

Asymptomatic bacteriuria is a clinical syndrome defined as the isolation of $\geq 10^5$ CFU/ml of bacteria from an appropriately collected clean urine specimen [69]. By definition, a positive culture of two urine specimens for the same bacteria is required in women, whereas a single urine culture is required in men [52].

Studies have shown a 4–7% prevalence of bacteriuria during pregnancy, compared to 1–3% prevalence in young nonpregnant women [70, 71]. Another risk population is diabetics over 70 years of age and those that use permanent or intermittent urinary catheters [72–75]. Screening and treatment of asymptomatic bacteriuria is only recommended in pregnant women, prior to prostate surgery or an invasive urological procedure [76]. Studies have shown a high prevalence of asymptomatic bacteriuria in HIV-infected pregnant women than among uninfected pregnant women [77–79]. In men infected with HIV/AIDS with a CD4 count <200, bacteriuria can reach up to 30% [36].

5. Etiology in different scenarios

UTIs in HIV patients are generally caused by the same gram-negative bacterial uropathogens that cause infections in healthy hosts, with *E. coli* being the predominant pathogen isolated. HIV status had no significant impact on the uropathogens that caused UTI in any setting [80]. However, the resistance of *E. coli* isolates demonstrated significantly higher resistance to co-trimoxazole compared to isolates from known HIV-negative patients (95% vs. 72%) (P: 0.001). Antimicrobial resistance has already emerged to most oral agents in the world including HIV- and non-HIV-infected patients.

Enterobacteriaceae, especially *E. coli*, is the major aerobic organism residing in the intestine and is the most reported cause of UTI [81, 82] being a common fecal contaminant, accounting for more than 60% of urinary isolates in HIV-infected patients. *Klebsiella*, *Enterococcus*, *Enterobacter*, and *Proteus* species are the next most common pathogens isolated [7, 22]. *Salmonella* and *Neisseria gonorrhoeae* can rarely cause prostatitis [42].

The exact etiology of UTIs is difficult to know. Most of the studies are retrospective in which clinical records or databases were analyzed. Many are already very old and have the limitation that the identification of the etiological agent is focused on bacteria, and routine tests are not included to identify other microorganisms such as fungi, parasites, and virus. In most centers, molecular DNA amplification tests were not used to identify organisms of fastidious growth. **Table 3** shows us the relevant information from selected studies on the etiology of UTIs in HIV-infected patients.

Reference author	**[83] Vignesh**	**[7] Schönwald**	**[84] Tessema**	**[85] Klapaczyńska**	**[86] Marami**
Year	2008	1999	2000	2018	2019
Country	India	Croatia	Esthiopia	Poland	Ethiopia
Analysis	Retrospective	Retrospective	Retrospective	Retrospective	A cross-sectional
N. patients	85	96	23	141	63
Female (%)	28.0	18.7	86.9	51.8	73.0
CD4 (cells/μl)	NA	NA	≥200 (74%)	139 (mean)	<200 (55.6%)
E. coli	42.3	22	69.6	82 (58.2)	24 (38.1)
S. aureus	21.2	0.0	8.7	1 (0.7)	7 (11.1)
K. pneumoniae	17.6	7.5	8.7	2 (1.4)	15 (23.8)

Reference author	[83] Vignesh	[7] Schönwald	[84] Tessema	[85] Klapaczyńska	[86] Marami
Enterococcus sp	8.2	26	0.0	18 (12.8)	2 (3.2)
Pseudomonas sp	3.5	15	4.3	5 (3.5)	4 (6.4)
Proteus sp	3.5	5.5	0.0	3 (2.1)	0.0
S. epidermidis	3.5	1.8	0.0	7 (5.0)	0.0
Other CONS*	0.0	0.0	0.0	3 (2.1)	5 (7.9)
Enterobacter sp	0.0	5.5	8.7	1 (0.7)	0.0
Acinctobacter sp	0.0	5.5	0.0	1 (0.7)	0.0
Providencia sp	0.0	3.7	0.0	0.0	0.0
S. agalactie	0.0	0.0	0.0	4 (2.8)	0.0
Streptococcus sp	0.0	0.0	0.0	3 (2.1)	0.0
C. albicans	0.0	0.0	0.0	1 (0.7)	0.0
S. emteritidis	0	1.8	0.0	0.0	0.0
S. maltophilia	0.0	0.0	0.0	1 (0.7)	0.0
M. morganii	0.0	0.0	0.0	1 (0.7)	0.0
Serratia odorifera	0.0	0.0	0.0	1 (0.7)	0.0
Sin cultivo	NA	NA	NA	NA	NA
Mixed patogen	0.0	0.0	0.0	4 (2.8)	0.0
Other	0.0	0.0	0.0	3 (2.1)	0.0

Coagulase-negative Staphylococci; ND = not done.

Table 3.
Studies showing the frequency of organisms causing UTIs in HIV infected patients.

5.1 Hospital-acquired UTIs

HIV-infected patients may be at a greater risk of HAI. In a study of 210 subjects, a rate of 15% of HAI was found in HIV-infected patients compared with only 6.9% of their overall nosocomial rates [65]. More than 75% of hospital-acquired UTIs are initiated by urinary catheters, which are used during the treatment of 15–25% of hospitalized patients. Common bacteria associated with CAUTI are *Staphylococcus aureus*, *E. coli*, *Pseudomonas aeruginosa*. *P. mirabilis*, *Staphylococcus epidermidis*, *Enterococcus faecalis*, and *Klebsiella pneumoniae* [57].

A retrospective cohort study [87] was carried out in an academic health system in New York City, which included 10,575 (697 UTIs) HIV-positive discharges from four hospitals over a period from 2006 to 2014. The rates of HAIs among HIV-infected patients are likely to be higher than those among HIV-uninfected patients; the risk factors were similar. The main organisms isolated in UTIs were *Acinetobacter baumannii*, *E. faecalis*, *K. pneumoniae*, *Pseudomonas aeruginosa*, and *Staphylococcus aureus*. Further research is required to address how patients' CD4 counts and viral loads affect their susceptibility to HAIs. Strategies to prevent nosocomial infections among HIV-infected patients are the same control measures used in HIV-uninfected patients [88].

In a Brazilian study, the overall incidence of HAIs was 5.90 per 1000 patient-days. The rates of HAI were 8.16 for HIV-positive and 3.94 for HIV-negative patients ($P = 0.01$). The most common HAIs were bloodstream infection in 44%, followed by UTIs with 18%, vascular infections in 14%, and pneumonia in 11%. Common etiologic agents were *A. baumanii*, *E. coli*, *E. faecalis*, *K pneumoniae*, *P. aeruginosa*, and yeast. Only three UTIs were detected in HIV-positive patients and 7 in HIV-negative patients [66].

5.2 AIDS with low CD4 count

HIV patients with a CD4 count <200 cells/μL are reported by some authors to be at a higher risk for UTIs, while others report that CD4 count is not associated with UTIs [36, 89, 90]. Few studies report the CD4 averages of patients with UTIs, and in some cases, etiology analysis is performed, separating patients with CD4 greater or less than 200 cells, in which no major differences have been reported in terms of isolated organisms. However, there are few reports of AIDS patients in very advanced stages, including some autopsy studies. In patients with AIDS, infections by atypical pathogens include fungi, parasites, mycobacteria, and viruses. These organisms are often widely disseminated at the time of urinary tract involvement and are usually associated with CD4 counts of $<100/mm^3$ [39, 91].

In patients with AIDS and disseminated *Cryptococcus neoformans* infection, prostate involvement may serve as a hidden site of persistent infection [92]. Fungal etiology is uncommon in immunocompromised and diabetic patients with chronic prostatitis [93].

The most illustrative study is by Miles et al. [19], which was carried out very early in the AIDS pandemic (1984–1987) in 120 patients, when there was still no antiretroviral treatment. They found a UTI prevalence of 14% (17 patients); only 9 had standard bacterial urinary infections. In the remaining 8 patients, 1 had gonorrhea, and 7 had positive urinary cultures that considered a manifestation of the systemic disease (6 with CMV and 1 with *Cryptococcus*). Autopsies were performed in 22 males and 1 female; the predominant urogenital finding was the absence and/or reduction of spermatogenesis in 17 patients. CMV was noted in the adrenal glands in 12 cases, one in bladder and prostate, respectively. Kaposi's sarcoma occurred in 4 cases. Numerous genitourinary sites involved with CMV and Kaposi's sarcoma suggested the systemic nature of these illnesses.

Renal tuberculosis has been detected in about 6–23% of AIDS patients by autopsy; a significant proportion of these cases were asymptomatic [42, 94, 95]. *Mycobacterium tuberculosis* is the most common species reported, followed by *Mycobacterium avium* and *Mycobacterium intracellulare*. Renal tuberculosis initially affects the kidney and by descending matter involves the ureters and lower urinary tract structures. When renal tuberculosis is suspected, polymerase chain reaction may be useful as a rapid assay to detect *M. tuberculosis*-specific DNA or RNA materials in urine [96, 97].

5.3 Asymptomatic HIV patients

A study with 317 asymptomatic HIV patients (89 men, 228 women), the prevalence of UTI did not differ significantly from those with a CD4 count less or high of 200 cells/μL. Females showed significantly higher prevalence of asymptomatic UTI than males [20]. The microbiology findings of urine culture are showed in **Table 4**, and the susceptibility of the isolated pathogens is showed in **Table 5**.

Organisms	**NonHIV (n = 104)**	**HAART naive (n = 101)**	**On HAART* (n = 216)**
Escherichia coli	6 (31.5)	4 (12.9)	6 (9.4)
Klebsiella species	0 (0.00)	1 (3.2)	5 (7.8)
Proteus species	0 (0.00)	1 (3.2	3 (4.7)
Staphylococcus aureus	6 (31.5)	8 (25.8)	17 (26.6)
Coagulase-negative Staphylococci	4 (21.5)	5 (16.1)	10 (15.6)
Enterococcus faecalis	0 (0.00)	1 (3.2)	8 (12.5)
Candida albicans	3 (15.8)	7 (22.6)	15 (23.4)
Trichomonas vaginalis	0 (0.00)	4 (12.9)	0 (0.00)
Total	19 (16.7)	31 (27.2)	64 (56.1)

**On HAART = ARVs use for three to six months.*
Modified from Omoregie and Eghafona [20].

Table 4.
Pathogens isolated from urine culture in asymptomatic HIV patients.

Antibacterial agents (µg/disc)	**Organisms**					
	***E. coli* (n = 16)**	***Klebsiella* sp. (n = 6)**	***Proteus* sp. (n = 4)**	***S. aureus* (n = 31**	**CONS* (n = 19)**	***E. faecalis* (n=9)**
Amoxicillin (30)	1 (6.2)	1 (16.7)	1 (25.0)	10 (32.2)	6 (31.6)	4 (44.4)
Amoxicillin/clav (30)	6 (6.2)	1 (16.7)	2 (50.0)	11 (35.5)	5 (26.3)	4 (44.4)
Gentamicin (10)	3 (18.7)	0 (0.0)	1 (25.0)	5 (16.1)	5 (26.3)	4 (44.4)
Co-trimoxazole (25)	1 (6.2)	1 (16.7)	0 (0.0)	1 (3.2)	1 (5.3)	0 (0.0)
Tetracycline (25)	0 (0.0)	0 (0.0)	0 (0.0)	1 (3.2)	0 (0.0)	1 (11.1)
Nitrofuratoin (300)	9 (56.2)	1 (16.7)	2 (50.0)	16 (51.6)	12 (63.2)	6 (66.7)
Nalidixic acid (30	3 (18.7)	0 (0.0)	0 (0.0)	ND	ND	ND
Ciprofloxacin (5)	6 (37.5)	2 (33.3)	2 (50.0)	10 (32.2)	8 (42.1)	5 (55.6)
Ofloxacin (5)	6 (37.5)	0 (0.0)	1 (25.0)	5 (16.1)	6 (31.6)	3 (33.3)

**Coagulase-negative* Staphylococci; *ND = not done.*
Adapted from Omoregie and Eghafona [20].

Table 5.
Susceptibility of bacterial isolates (number and percent).

6. Susceptibility drugs and therapy

Bacterial resistance is a major public health problem, which mainly affects developing countries. The irrational and indiscriminate use of antibiotics and deficient surveillance programs on antibiotic use are common in these countries [98, 99]. According to the etiological tendency, clinicians should know these changes for effective treatment of UTIs and to avoid antibiotic misuse.

In a recent study in Southern Ethiopia [84] of 224 study participants, bacteria have been isolated from 23 patients, 11 (4.9%) with symptomatic and 12 (5.4%) with asymptomatic UTI; most of participants were females (58.5%). Twenty-one (91.3%)

Antibacterial agents (μg/disc)	Organisms				
	E. coli (n = 16)	*K. pneumoniae* (n=2)	*E. aurogenes* (n = 2)	*Pseudomonas* spp. (n = 1)	*S. aureus* (n = 2)
Ampicillin	0 (0.0)	0 (0.0)	0 (0.0)	0 (0.0)	NA
Ciprofloxacin (30)	14 (87.5)	2 (100)	2 (100)	1 (100)	2 (100)
Cotrimoxazole (30)	6 (37.5)	2 (100)	1 (50)	0 (0.0)	0 (0.0)
Gentamicin (10)	15 (93.8)	2 (100)	2 (100)	1 (100)	2 (100)
Meropenem (25)	14 (87.5)	2 (100)	2 (100)	1 (100)	NA
Nitrofuratoin (300)	16 (100)	2 (100)	2 (100)	0 (0.0)	2 (100)
Amoxicillin/clav	11 (68.8)	0 (0.0)	1 (50)	1 (100)	NA
Cefriaxone	16 (100)	1 (50)	1 (50)	1 (100)	NA
Norfloxacin	14 (87.5)	2 (100)	2 (100)	0 (0.0)	2 (100)
Ceftazidime	8 (50)	2 (100)	1 (50)	1 (100)	NA
Tetracycline	5 (31.3)	1 (50)	1 (50)	0 (0.0)	0 (0.0)
Clindamycin	NA	NA	NA	NA	2 (100)
penicillin	NA	NA	NA	NA	2 (100)
erythromycin	NA	NA	NA	NA	2 (100)
Cefoxitin	NA	NA	NA	NA	2 (100)

Modified from Tessema et al. [84].

Table 6.
Susceptibility of bacterial isolates from UTIs of HIV infected patients (number and percent).

of isolates were gram-negative bacteria where *E. coli* was the most predominant isolate. Drug testing was done by the Kirby-Bauer disk diffusion method; susceptibility findings are shown in **Table 6**. Most of the bacterial isolates were susceptible to ciprofloxacin, ceftriaxone, gentamicin, nitrofurantoin, and norfloxacin. The isolates were resistant to ampicillin, tetracycline, and co-trimoxazole. Multidrug resistant bacteria were common in this study [84].

In another study published in 2019, *E. coli* was resistant to ampicillin (95.8%), ceftazidime (95.8%), cotrimoxazole (95.8%), amoxicillin (91.7%), ceftriaxone (87.5%), and tetracycline (87.2%); 46% were multidrug resistant. On other hand, *E. coli* and the rest of the gram-negative bacilli were sensitive to quinolones (ciprofloxacin, norfloxacin) as well as gentamicin in about 75%. *S. aureus* exhibited a high proportion of resistance (85.7%) to each of ampicillin, amoxicillin, and cotrimoxazole. Coagulase-negative *Staphylococcus* were 100% resistant to each of ampicillin and amoxicillin and 80% to chloramphenicol. However, it is important to note that antibiotics such as carbapenems, piperacillin tazobactam, tigecycline, and other new antibiotics were not tested for gram-negative bacteria and that third-generation cephalosporins, vancomycin, linezolid, and tigecycline were also not tested for gram-positive bacteria [86].

E. coli isolates from known HIV-positive patients demonstrated significantly higher resistance to co-trimoxazole. HIV status did not affect resistance patterns to the other antimicrobials that were examined. Resistance of *E. coli* to ampicillin and co-trimoxazole was greater than 60%; authors recommended that these agents should not be used as empiric treatment for UTI. Additionally, given that there was greater than

20% resistance to ciprofloxacin, its use would otherwise be inappropriate as an empiric agent in the context of Botswana [80].

6.1 Treatment of UTIs in HIV infected patients

Like the general population, the treatment of UTIs should be individualized; in patients with AIDS, a culture-specific treatment is recommended. To select a specific treatment, it is advisable to follow the international treatment guidelines. It is recommended that the guidelines be recent [100, 101], according to how the epidemiology of UTIs and resistance evolve in specific populations. Despite clear guidelines, practice patterns vary widely with numerous studies showing substantial discrepancies between clinical practice guidelines and antibiotic-prescribing practices [102].

In the selection of empirical therapy of UTIs, it is necessary to define if the patient had some risk factor for complicated UTI. The evidence suggests that HIV-infected patients had the same or almost the same behavior as non-infected HIV population. Microbiology studies show that enterebocateriaceae, especially *E. coli*, are primarily implicated. This may apply to different populations of HIV patients, including the most common complicated UTIs, such as hospital-acquired UTIs, associated or not with the use of a urinary catheter, pregnant patients, elderly patients, and in cases of asymptomatic bacteriuria.

On recent guidelines [100] for urological infections, the following tables show the suggested therapy for different scenarios: Uncomplicated cystitis (**Table 7**), uncomplicated pyelonephritis (**Table 8**), parenteral antimicrobial therapy in uncomplicated pyelonephritis (**Table 9**), urosepsis (**Table 10**), and chronic bacterial prostatitis (**Table 11**).

The diagnostic approach varies according to clinical suspicion; at best, a general urine examination accompanied by a urinary culture with antimicrobial sensitivity tests is reasonably chosen for its already recognized activity against urinary pathogens. Many sites are using obsolete panels containing useless antimicrobial agents such as tetracyclines, chloramphenicol, and others, without the new useful antimicrobial

Antimicrobial	Daily dose	Duration of therapy	Comments
First-line women			
Fosfomycin trometamol	3 g SD	1 day	Recommended only in women with uncomplicated cystitis
Nitrofurantoin macrocrystal	50–100 mg	5 days	
Nitrofurantoin monohydrate/ macrocrystals	100 mg b.i.d.	5 days	
Nitrofurantoin macrocrystal prolonged release	100 mg b.i.d.	5 days	
Pivmecillinam	400 mg t.i.d.	3–5 days	
Alternatives			
Cephalosporins (e.g. cefadroxil)	500 mg b.i.d.	3 days	Or comparable
If the local resistance pattern for *E. coli* is < 20%			
Trimethoprim	200 mg b.i.d.	5 days	Not in the first trimenon of pregnancy
Trimethoprimsulfamethoxazole	160/800 mg b.i.d.	3 days	Not in the last trimenon of pregnancy

Antimicrobial	Daily dose	Duration of therapy	Comments
Treatment in men			
Trimethoprim/ sulfamethoxazole	160/800 mg b.i.d.	7 days	Fluoroquinolones can also be prescribed in accordance with local susceptibility testing.

SD = single dose; b.i.d. = twice daily; t.i.d. = three times daily.
Adapted from Bonkat et al. [100].

Table 7.
Suggested regimens for antimicrobial therapy in uncomplicated cystitis.

Antimicrobial	Daily dose	Duration of therapy	Comments
Ciprofloxacin	500–750 mg b.i.d.	7 days	Fluoroquinolone resistance should be less than 10%
Levofloxacin	750 mg q.d.	5 days	
Trimethoprim sulfamethoxazol	160/800 mg b.i.d.	14 days	If such agents are used empirically, an initial intravenous dose of a long-acting parenteral antimicrobial (e.g. ceftriaxone) should be administered
Cefpodoxime	200 mg b.i.d.	10 days	
Ceftibuten	400 mg q.d.	10 days	

b.i.d. = twice daily; q.d. = every day.
Adapted from Bonkat et al. [100].

Table 8.
Suggested regimens for empirical oral antimicrobial therapy in uncomplicated pyelonephritis.

Antimicrobials	Daily dose	Comments
First-line treatment		
Ciprofloxacin	400 mg b.i.d.	
Levofloxacin	750 mg q.d	
Cefotaxime	2 g t.i.d.	Not studied as monotherapy in acute uncomplicated pyelonephritis.
Ceftriaxone	1–2 g q.d.	Lower dose studied, but higher dose recommended.
Second-line treatment		
Cefepime	1–2 g b.i.d.	Lower dose studied, but higher dose recommended
Piperacillin/ tazobactam	2.5–4.5 g t.i.d.	
Gentamicin	5 mg/kg q.d.	Not studied as monotherapy in acute uncomplicated pyelonephritis.
Amikacin	15 mg/kg q.d.	
Last-line alternatives		
Imipenem/ cilastatin	0.5 g t.i.d.	Consider only in patients with early culture results indicating the presence of multi-drug resistant organisms.
Meropenem	1 g t.i.d.	
Ceftolozane/ tazobactam	1.5 g t.i.d.	

Antimicrobials	Daily dose	Comments
Ceftazidime/ avibactam	2.5 g t.i.d.	
Cefiderocol	2 g t.i.d.	
Meropenem-vaborbactam	2 g t.i.d.	
Plazomicin	15 mg/kg o.d.	

b.i.d. = twice daily; t.i.d. = three times daily; q.d. = every day; o.d. = once daily.
Adapted from Bonkat et al. [100].

Table 9.
Suggested regimens for empirical parenteral antimicrobial therapy in uncomplicated pyelonephritis.

Antimicrobials	Daily dose	Duration of therapy
Cefotaxime	2 g t.i.d.	7–10 days Longer courses are appropriate in patients who have a slow clinical response
Ceftazidime	1–2 g t.i.d.	
Ceftriaxone	1–2 g q.d.	
Cefepime	2 g b.i.d.	
Piperacillin/ tazobactam	4.5 g t.i.d.	
Ceftolozane/ tazobactam	1.5 g t.i.d.	
Ceftazidime/ avibactam	2.5 g t.i.d.	
Gentamicin*	5 mg/kg q.d.	
Amikacin*	15 mg/kg q.d.	
Ertapenem	1 g q.d.	
Imipenem/ cilastatin	0.5 g t.i.d.	
Meropenem	1 g t.i.d.	

**Not studied as monotherapy in urosepsis, b.i.d. = twice daily; t.i.d. = three times daily; q.d. = every day.*
Adapted from Bonkat et al. [100].

Table 10.
Suggested regimens for antimicrobial therapy for urosepsis.

Antimicrobial	Daily dose	Duration of therapy	Comments
Floroquinolone	Optimal oral daily dose	4–6 weeks	
Doxycycline	100 mg b.i.d	10 days	Only for *C. trachomatis* or *Mycoplasma* infections
Azithromycin	500 mg once daily	3 weeks	Only for *C. trachomatis* infections

Antimicrobial	Daily dose	Duration of therapy	Comments
Metronidazole	500 mg t.i.d.	14 days	Only for *T. vaginalis* infections

b.i.d. = twice daily; t.i.d. = three times daily.
Adapted from Bonkat et al. [100].

Table 11.
Suggested regimens for antimicrobial therapy for chronic bacterial prostatitis.

agents. It is not uncommon that in a culture where an *Acinectobacter baumannii* grows, sensitivity to antibiotics such as colistin and tigecycline is not included in the report. The laboratory and the medical engineers who manufacture part of these supplies should also be advised about these queries.

Patients with complicated infections or recurrent infections, both infected or not by HIV, require additional studies that in many cases are aimed to find the cause of the recurrence; sometimes, it can be obvious such as pregnancy or the use of urinary catheter. Other factors for recurrence of UTIs such as malformations of the urinary tract, bladder ureter reflux, retentionist bladder, and the presence of a tumor or lithiasis are usually not in sight and require additional diagnostic tests such as plain film of the abdomen, ultrasonography, computed tomography, magnetic resonance, and cystography to detect correctable structural or functional abnormalities. Urodynamic findings in HIV patients included acontractile hypoactive bladder and detrusor-sphincter dyssynergia [4]. In patients with urinary retention, hypocontractility of the bladder was observed in 35–45% and prostatic enlargement in only 18%. Many of these patients required intermittent catheterization [103].

6.2 Treatment of UTIs for non-bacterial causes

Patients with AIDS, especially those with <100 CD4 cells/mm^3, the etiology of UTIs may be related to the spread of infections; the etiological agents may be diverse as they have already been described in this population [9, 42]. These patients require cultures and sensitivity tests not only for bacteria but also for cultures and stains for fungi and mycobacteria. Parasites should be searched, and molecular tests should include viruses such as CMV and adenovirus; GeneXpert for *M. tuberculosis,* which is a widespread test, is accessible and with high diagnostic value. The diagnostic approach may also vary according to the microbial epidemiology of each country and the accessibility of diagnostic tests. Fungal pathogens are related to a weakened immune system due to diseases such as HIV, cancer, organ transplantation, or by the use of certain drugs, resulting in the body's inability to fight infection. Long-term use of antifungal drugs can easily lead to fungal resistance; more than 90% of fungus-related deaths are caused by *Cryptococcus*, *Candida*, *Aspergillus*, *Histoplasma*, and *Pneumocystis* [104].

To choose the treatment in cases of UTIs by a fungal pathogen, it is necessary to have knowledge of the various therapeutic options, especially some pharmacological principles about the spectrum of antifungals, the safety of their use, and the possibility of resistance. Hospital-acquired UTIs and overall those associated with long-term urinary catheter use in AIDS patients with very low CD4 counts have a high risk for *Candida* and other fungi UTIs [105]. **Figure 1** shows the current antifungals and their modes of action, and **Table 12** shows the generalities about the spectrum of antifungal agents by family.

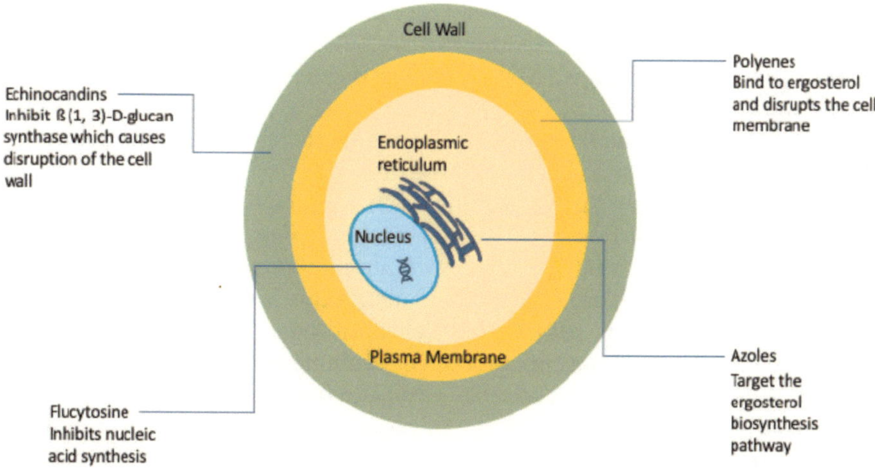

Figure 1.
Simplified schematic diagram depicting the current antifungals and their modes of action. Adapted with permission from: Wall and Lopez-Ribot [105].

Antifungal class	Biological effect	Spectrum of action
Polyenes	Fungicidal	Broad spectrum antifungal in treatment of invasive fungal infections; resistance is rare.
Flucytosine	Fungicidal against *Cryptococcus* spp.	Almost exclusively used for cryptococcal meningitis, but resistance is extremely common so never used in monotherapy.
Azoles	Mostly fungistatic	As a class they display broad spectrum against yeasts and filamentous fungi, although some species display intrinsic resistance to commonly used derivatives; secondary resistance can often develop during treatment.
Echinocandins	Fungicidal against *Candida* spp., but fungistatic against *Aspergillus* spp.	First line of defense for candidiasis and used in aspergillosis when refractory to other treatments; resistance is emerging.

Modified from: Wall and Lopez-Ribot [105].

Table 12.
Agent classes for the treatment of invasive fungal infections.

Candida UTI can be caused by a hematogenous spread following candidemia or by retrograde route via the urethra. Fluconazole is the treatment of choice for symptomatic infections, having a high urine concentration. Other antifungal azoles and echinocandins do not reach sufficient urinary levels. Amphotericin B deoxycholate (AmB) is the recommended therapy in cases of intolerance or resistance to fluconazole. **Table 12** shows the treatment of UTIs caused by Candida species [106].

In 1990, Fluconazole became available and is now the most used azole for systemic fungal infections, particularly those caused by yeast (i.e., *Candida*, *Cryptococcus*). Emerging fungi such as *Aspergillus* show intrinsic resistance to fluconazole, requiring the use of itraconazole or voriconazole. Mucorales are another group of aggressive fungi that cause systemic infections and for which posaconazole and more recently isavuconazole have been used. Azole resistance is common during treatment due to various mechanisms, including mutations in the ERG11 target gene and overexpression of efflux pumps [107]. Despite resistance, azoles are still some of the most used antifungal drugs.

Fluconazole is one of the few antifungals with a good elimination by urine, reaching a concentration of about 80% of the drug in unchanged form. The use of fluconazole may have some limitations due to drug interactions, liver toxicity, QT prolongation, and resistance of some non-*Candida albicans* species such as *C. glabrata* and *C. krusei*. Treatment of *C. glabrata* infections may require high doses (800 mg/day) or definitive use of AmB as an alternative if the isolate is highly resistant to fluconazole [108, 109]. Other azole antifungals are poorly eliminated in the urine, which limits their use in cystitis. For example, itraconazole achieves a concentration of only <1%, voriconazole <5%, and posaconazole <1% [110]. Isavuconazole also has negligible urinary excretion and is unlikely to be useful for the treatment of UTIs [111]. Posaconazole and voriconazole are well concentrated in renal tissue and may be effective in the treatment of *Candida* pyelonephritis [110]. The echinocandins (caspofungin, anidulafungin, and micafungin) are only <2% concentrated in urine, so they are not recommended for the treatment of lower urinary tract infections, but they can reach high concentrations in the renal parenchyma [112]. There are some reports of cases that were successfully treated with echinocandins as rescue in complicated UTIs [113–115]. Caspofungin was the first echinocandin to be approved for use in humans in 2001; subsequently, two other echinocandins (micafungin in 2005 and anidulafungin in 2006) were approved [116, 117]. As a consequence of increased drug exposure, there has been an increase in the development of resistance mostly in strains different to *C. albicans* [116].

The major problem with amB has always been its toxicity presenting itself as chills, fever, dyspnea, hypokalemia, and nephrotoxicity that can lead to kidney failure. Thus, several lipid formulations of amB, including liposomal amB, amB lipid complex, and amB colloidal dispersion, have been developed, which generally show decreased toxicity and improved pharmacokinetic parameters that depend to a large extent on the composition and particle size of the nanoformulations [118]. The Infectious Diseases Society of America (IDSA) recommends deoxycholate AmB but not lipid formulations for the treatment of Candida UTI [109, 112].

Reactivation of latent CMV infection (usually acquired during childhood) occurs in >40% of patients with AIDS. UTI caused by CMV is often asymptomatic, but rare cases of symptomatic CMV cystitis have been reported; antiviral agents, for example, ganciclovir or foscarnet, can be necessary in the treatment of this disease [19, 42]. In 1989, ganciclovir became the first anti-CMV agent approved by the US Food and Drug Administration for the treatment and prevention of CMV infection and disease, followed by foscarnet, cidofovir, and valganciclovir. New agents with a novel mechanism of action such as letermovir and possibly maribavir are brought to clinical use; combination therapy for the treatment of CMV infection and disease becomes, for the first time, a possibility, especially in serious clinical presentations [119].

Treatment of tuberculosis in HIV-infected patients represents great challenges. Drug interactions and adverse events must always be taken as a risk, and a close monitoring must be carried out to avoid complications and clinical worsening. Per se, the standard (first-line) anti-TB therapy is already associated with adverse events and even intolerance. The interaction between rifampicin and many ARV drugs requires adjustment from a standard ARV regimen to a modified one. In addition, there is a risk of developing resistance when tuberculosis is treated using intermittent therapy.

The treatment recommendation for HIV-infected patients receiving ARVs who have drug-sensitive tuberculosis consists of a 6-month regimen, of which during the first 2 months (intensive phase), 4 drugs are given daily: isoniazid (INH), rifampicin (RIF), pyrazinamide (PZA), and ethambutol (EMB), which is usually given as compacted tablets that are calculated by weight. In the continuation phase, only two drugs (INH and RIF) are used and are administered every third day for 4 months. In the rare situation where HIV-infected patients do not receive ART during TB treatment, the recommendation is to extend the continuation phase with INH and RIF for an additional 3 months (i.e., a continuation phase of 7 months in duration, corresponding to a total of 9 months of therapy) [120]. Pyridoxine (vitamin B6) is given with INH to all persons at risk of neuropathy (e.g., pregnant women; breastfed infants; persons infected with HIV; patients with diabetes, alcoholism, malnutrition, or chronic renal failure; or those who are of advanced age) [121, 122].

The use of intermittent tuberculosis treatment regimens in HIV-infected patients has been associated with high rates of relapse and the emergence of drug resistance [123, 124]. Relapse and resistance were associated with low CD4 lymphocyte counts, as all recurrences occurred in patients with baseline CD4 lymphocyte counts of <100 cells/μL. Lower plasma concentrations of rifabutin and INH were identified as key risk factors for acquiring rifamycin resistance [125]. ART should ideally be started within 2 weeks for those patients with a CD4 count of <50 cells/μL and by 8–12 weeks for those with a CD4 count of ≥50 cells/μL [126]. The concurrent administration of ARV and rifamycin is a major therapeutic challenge. RIF can modify the concentration of some drugs in the treatment of HIV infection, especially protease and integrase inhibitors [127, 128].

Late-stage HIV patients with CD4+ cell counts of <50 cells/μL who initiate ARV therapy are at high risk of developing immune reconstitution inflammatory syndrome (IRIS) [129]. IRIS can present with high fever and generalized lymphadenopathy or with localized manifestations including respiratory symptoms, infiltrates or pleural effusions, abdominal pain, retroperitoneal abscesses, headache, seizures, and focal neurological deficits. M. tuberculosis, Toxoplasma, P. jirovecii, and *C. neoformans* are the main pathogens involved [130]. For more severe cases of IRIS, treatment with corticosteroids is effective. In a placebo-controlled trial of prednisone for patients with moderate IRIS, prednisone 1.25 mg/kg/day significantly reduced the need for hospitalization or surgical procedures [131].

7. Conclusion

UTI is considered the most common bacterial infection, mainly affecting women. From 15 to 50 years of age, UTI is practically nonexistent in men, but in those older than 65 years, the prevalence of bacteriuria and UTI increases substantially in men to almost equal that of elderly women. The prevalence of hospital-acquired UTI increases significantly in AIDS patients, mainly in patients with <200 CD4 cells/mm^3. Asymptomatic bacteriuria is more prevalent in HIV-infected pregnant women than among uninfected pregnant women. Bacteriuria can reach up to 30% in AIDS patients.

A specific risk factor for UTI can be present, including sexual activity, pregnancy, indwelling catheter drainage, neurogenic bladder, prostatism, and urethral stricture, among many others. Some of these risk factors can be inferred from proper questioning. There is a consensus that people with lower CD4 have a high risk of developing UTIs as well as other opportunistic infections. However, it is unclear whether HIV/AIDS imposes an additional risk for UTI.

UTIs in HIV patients are generally caused by the same gram-negative bacteria that cause infections in healthy hosts, with *E. coli* being the predominant pathogen isolated. *Klebsiella*, *Enterococcus*, *Enterobacter*, and *Proteus* species are the next most common pathogens isolated. In AIDS patients, especially those with <100 CD4 cells/mm^3, the etiology of UTIs may be diverse and associated with disseminated infections by atypical pathogens including CMV, adenovirus, *Cryptococcus*, *Candida*, *M. tuberculosis*, and Kaposi's sarcoma. **Figure 2** summarizes the most relevant aspects of this chapter.

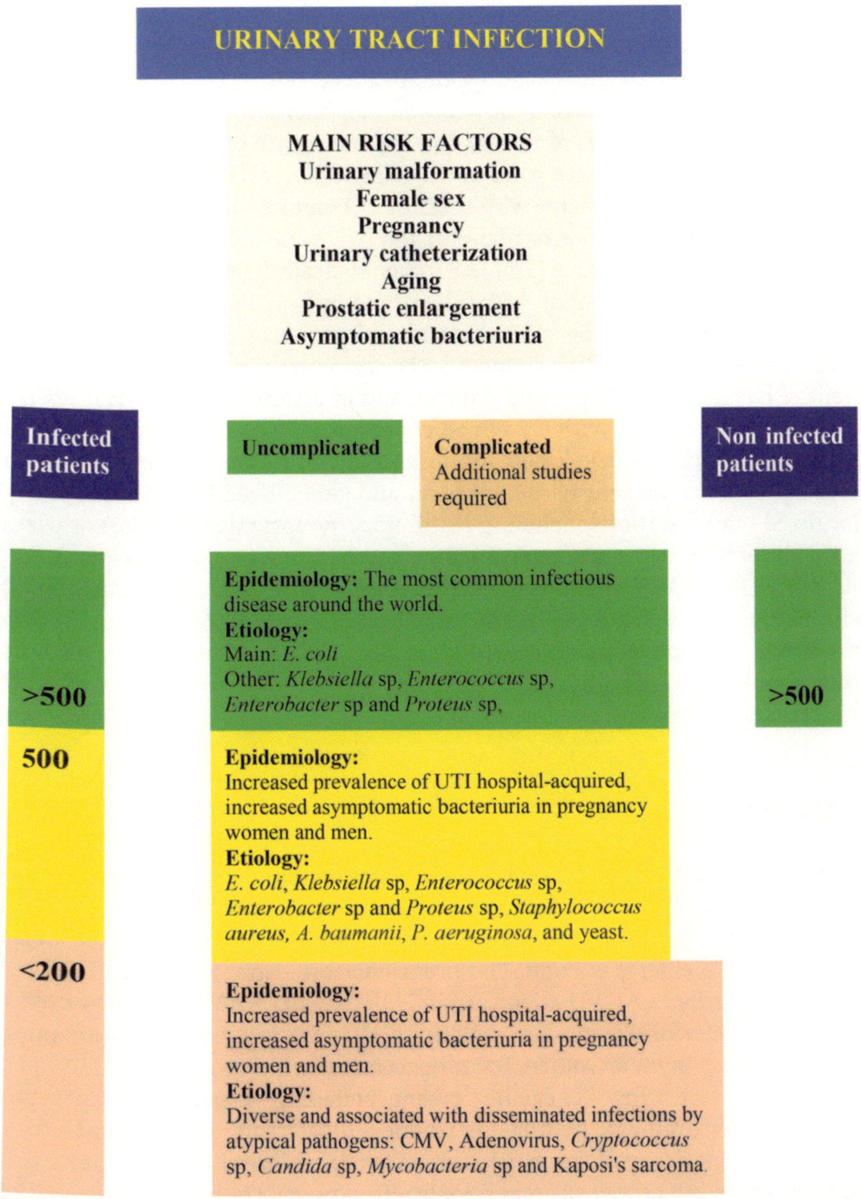

Figure 2.
Summary of the most relevant features of UTI in HIV/AIDS patients.

The diagnostic approach may also vary according to the microbial epidemiology of each country and the accessibility of diagnostic tests such as molecular techniques. Like the general population, the treatment of UTIs should be individualized; an etiology determination is recommended in AIDS patients in order to select a specific treatment; it is advisable to follow the international treatment guidelines.

Acknowledgements

We offer particular thanks to *Karen I. Amaya Aguirre* (candidate in Pharmacological Research at Georgetown University) for the review of the manuscript and her valuable comments.

Funding sources

This research did not receive any specific grant from funding agencies in the public, commercial, or not-for-profit sectors.

Conflict of interest statement

The authors declare no conflicts of interest.

Author details

Gerardo Amaya-Tapia[1,2]*, Gabriela Ibarra-Nieto[2], Octavio Campollo Rivas[1,3] and José Luis González Sánchez[4]

1 Department of Medical Clinics, Universidad de Guadalajara, Mexico

2 Infectious Diseases Department, Hospital General de Occidente, Mexico

3 Center of Studies on Alcohol and Addictions, Antiguo Hospital Civil de Guadalajara, Mexico

4 Medicine Student, University Center of Health Sciences. Universidad de Guadalajara, Mexico

*Address all correspondence to: gerardo.amaya@academicos.udg.mx

References

[1] Foxman B. Epidemiology of urinary tract infections: Incidence, morbidity, and economic costs. The American Journal of Medicine. 2002;**113**(Suppl. 1A):5S-13S. DOI: 10.1016/s0002-9343(02)01054-9

[2] González-Chamorro F, Palacios R, Alcover J, Campos J, Borrego F, Dámaso D. La infección urinaria y su prevención [Urinary tract infections and their prevention]. Actas Urológicas Españolas. 2012;**36**(1):48-53. DOI: 10.1016/j.acuro.2011.05.002. Spanish. Epub 2011 Jul 14

[3] Foxman B, Barlow R, D'Arcy H, Gillespie B, Sobel JD. Urinary tract infection: Self-reported incidence and associated costs. Annals of Epidemiology. 2000;**10**(8):509-515. DOI: 10.1016/s1047-2797(00)00072-7

[4] Hermieu JF, Delmas V, Boccon-Gibod L. Micturition disturbances and human immunodeficiency virus infection. The Journal of Urology. 1996; **156**(1):157-159

[5] Kane CJ, Bolton DM, Connolly JA, Tanagho EA. Voiding dysfunction in human immunodeficiency virus infections. The Journal of Urology. 1996; **155**(2):523-526

[6] Asharam K, Bhimma R, Adhikari M. Human immunodeficiency virus and urinary tract infections in children. Annals of Tropical Paediatrics. 2003; **23**(4):273-277. DOI: 10.1179/027249303225007653

[7] Schönwald S, Begovac J, Skerk V. Urinary tract infections in HIV disease. International Journal of Antimicrobial Agents. 1999;**11**(3–4): 309-311. DOI: 10.1016/s0924-8579(99)00036-9

[8] Steele BW, Carson CC. Recognizing the urologic manifestations of HIV and AIDS. Contemporary Urology. 1997;**9**: 39-53

[9] Kaplan MS, Wechsler M, Benson MC. Urologic manifestations of AIDS. Urology. 1987;**30**(5):441-443. DOI: 10.1016/0090-4295(87)90375-x

[10] O'Regan S, Russo P, Lapointe N, Rousseau E. AIDS and the urinary tract. Journal of Acquired Immune Deficiency Syndromes (1988). 1990;3(3):244-251

[11] Nicolle LE. The prevention of hospital-acquired urinary tract infection. Clinical Infectious Diseases. 2008;**46**(2): 251-253. DOI: 10.1086/524663

[12] Tambyah PA, Maki DG. Catheter-associated urinary tract infection is rarely symptomatic: A prospective study of 1,497 catheterized patients. Archives of Internal Medicine. 2000;**160**(5):678-682. DOI: 10.1001/archinte.160.5.678

[13] Hooton TM, Bradley SF, Cardenas DD, Colgan R, Geerlings SE, Rice JC, et al. Diagnosis, prevention, and treatment of catheter-associated urinary tract infection in adults: 2009 International Clinical Practice Guidelines from the Infectious Diseases Society of America. Clinical Infectious Diseases. 2010;**50**(5):625-663. DOI: 10.1086/650482

[14] Foxman B. Urinary tract infection syndromes: Occurrence, recurrence, bacteriology, risk factors, and disease burden. Infectious Disease Clinics of North America. 2014;**28**(1):1-13. DOI: 10.1016/j.idc.2013.09.003. Epub 2013 Dec 8

[15] Abelson B, Sun D, Que L, Nebel RA, Baker D, Popiel P, et al. Sex differences

in lower urinary tract biology and physiology. Biology of Sex Differences. 2018;**9**(1):45. DOI: 10.1186/s13293-018-0204-8

[16] Ruben FL, Dearwater SR, Norden CW, Kuller LH, Gartner K, Shalley A, et al. Clinical infections in the noninstitutionalized geriatric age group: Methods utilized and incidence of infections. The Pittsburgh Good Health Study. of Epidemiology. 1995;**141**(2): 145-157. DOI: 10.1093/oxfordjournals.aje.a117402

[17] Harper M, Fowlis G. Management of urinary tract infections in men. Trends in Urology, Gynecology and Sexual Health. 2007;**12**:30-35. DOI: 10.1002/tre.8

[18] In Danger: UNAIDS Global AIDS Update 2022. Geneva: Joint United Nations Programme on HIV/AIDS; 2022. Licence: CC BY-NC-SA 3.0 IGO

[19] Miles BJ, Melser M, Farah R, Markowitz N, Fisher E. The urological manifestations of the acquired immunodeficiency syndrome. The Journal of Urology. 1989;**142**(3):771-773. DOI: 10.1016/s0022-5347(17)38883-3

[20] Omoregie R, Eghafona NO. Urinary tract infection among asymptomatic HIV patients in Benin City, Nigeria. British Journal of Biomedical Science. 2009; **66**(4):190-193. DOI: 10.1080/09674845.2009. 11730272

[21] De Pinho AM, Lopes GS, Ramos-Filho CF, Santos Oda R, De Oliveira MP, Halpern M, et al. Urinary tract infection in men with AIDS. Genitourinary Medicine. 1994;**70**(1):30-34. DOI: 10.1136/sti.70.1.30

[22] Yepes A, Ávila E, Carreño H, Barreto J, Currea IY, Chaves ES, et al. Prevalencia de la infección urinaria adquirida en la comunidad en pacientes con HIV/SIDA. RFS Revista Facultad de Salud. 2010;**2**(1):71-75. DOI: 10.25054/rfs.v2i1.91

[23] Boaitey YA, Nkrumah B, Idriss A, Tay SC. Gastrointestinal and urinary tract pathogenic infections among HIV seropositive patients at the Komfo Anokye Teaching Hospital in Ghana. BMC Research Notes. 2012;**5**:454. DOI: 10.1186/1756-0500-5-454

[24] Mota Loor AA, Palacios Aguirre ME, Ávalos Layana MA, Narea Morales VE. Infecciones urinarias asociadas a pacientes con VIH-sida. Pro Sciences: Revista De Producción, Ciencias E Investigación. 2022;**6**(43):176-182. DOI: 10.29018/issn.2588-1000vol6iss43.2022pp176-182

[25] Birhanu MY, Habtegiorgis SD, Gietaneh W, Alemu S, Tsegaye TB, Bekele GM, et al. Magnitude and associated factors of urinary tract infections among adults living with HIV in Ethiopia. Systematic review and meta-analysis. PLoS One. 2022;**17**(4): e0264732. DOI: 10.1371/journal.pone.0264732

[26] Ingersoll MA. Sex differences shape the response to infectious diseases. PLoS Pathogens. 2017;**13**(12):e1006688. DOI: 10.1371/journal.ppat.1006688

[27] Levison ME, Kaye D. Treatment of complicated urinary tract infections with an emphasis on drug-resistant gram-negative uropathogens. Current Infectious Disease Reports. 2013;**15**(2): 109-115. DOI: 10.1007/s11908-013-0315-7

[28] Lichtenberger P, Hooton TM. Complicated urinary tract infections. Current Infectious Disease Reports. 2008;**10**(6):499-504. DOI: 10.1007/s11908-008-0081-0

[29] Sleator RD. The human superorganism - of microbes and men. Medical Hypotheses. 2010;**74**(2): 214-215. DOI: 10.1016/j.mehy.2009. 08.047

[30] Culligan EP, Sleator RD, Marchesi JR, Hill C. Metagenomics and novel gene discovery: Promise and potential for novel therapeutics. Virulence. 2014;**5**(3):399-412. DOI: 10.4161/viru.27208. Epub 2013 Apr 1

[31] Vagios S, Hesham H, Mitchell C. Understanding the potential of lactobacilli in recurrent UTI prevention. Microbial Pathogenesis. 2020;**148**: 104544. DOI: 10.1016/j.micpath.2020. 104544. Epub 2020 Oct 1

[32] Gottschick C, Deng ZL, Vital M, Masur C, Abels C, Pieper DH, et al. The urinary microbiota of men and women and its changes in women during bacterial vaginosis and antibiotic treatment. Microbiome. 2017;**5**(1):99. DOI: 10.1186/s40168-017-0305-3

[33] Hilt EE, McKinley K, Pearce MM, Rosenfeld AB, Zilliox MJ, Mueller ER, et al. Urine is not sterile: Use of enhanced urine culture techniques to detect resident bacterial flora in the adult female bladder. Journal of Clinical Microbiology. 2014;**52**(3):871-876. DOI: 10.1128/JCM.02876-13. Epub 2013 Dec 26

[34] Croxen MA, Finlay BB. Molecular mechanisms of *Escherichia coli* pathogenicity. Nature Reviews. Microbiology 2010;8(1):26-38. doi: 10.1038/nrmicro2265. Erratum in: Nature Reviews. Microbiology 2013; **11**(2):141

[35] Johnson JR, Russo TA. Molecular epidemiology of extraintestinal pathogenic (uropathogenic) Escherichia coli. International Journal of Medical Microbiology. 2005;**295**(6–7):383-404. DOI: 10.1016/j.ijmm.2005.07.005

[36] Hoepelman AI, van Buren M, van den Broek J, Borleffs JC. Bacteriuria in men infected with HIV-1 is related to their immune status (CD4+ cell count). AIDS. 1992;**6**(2):179-184. DOI: 10.1097/ 00002030-199202000-00006

[37] Kwan DJ, Lowe FC. Acquired immunodeficiency syndrome. A venereal disease. The Urologic Clinics of North America. 1992;**19**(1):13-24

[38] Hyun G, Lowe FC. AIDS and the urologist. The Urologic Clinics of North America. 2003;**30**(1):101-109. DOI: 10.1016/s0094-0143(02)00124-6

[39] Wong JK, Yukl SA. Tissue reservoirs of HIV. Current Opinion in HIV and AIDS. 2016;**11**(4):362-370. DOI: 10.1097/ COH.0000000000000293

[40] Cohen MS, Shaw GM, McMichael AJ, Haynes BF. Acute HIV-1 infection. The New England Journal of Medicine. 2011;**364**(20):1943-1954. DOI: 10.1056/NEJMra1011874

[41] Scholz EMB, Kashuba ADM. The lymph node reservoir: Physiology, HIV infection, and antiretroviral therapy. Clinical Pharmacology and Therapeutics. 2021;**109**(4):918-927. DOI: 10.1002/ cpt.2186.Epub 2021 Feb 28

[42] Lee LK, Dinneen MD, Ahmad S. The urologist and the patient infected with human immunodeficiency virus or with acquired immunodeficiency syndrome. BJU International. 2001;**88**(6):500-510. DOI: 10.1046/j.1464-410x.2001.02376.x

[43] Itani S, Bartlett JA. Strategies of antiretroviral therapy in adults. The Urologic Clinics of North America. 1999;

26(4):809-820, ix-x. DOI: 10.1016/s0094-0143(05)70221-4

[44] Cihlar T, Fordyce M. Current status and prospects of HIV treatment. Current Opinion in Virology. 2016;**18**:50-56. DOI: 10.1016/j.coviro.2016.03.004. Epub 2016 Mar 28

[45] Guaraldi G, Orlando G, Zona S, Menozzi M, Carli F, Garlassi E, et al. Premature age-related comorbidities among HIV-infected persons compared with the general population. Clinical Infectious Diseases. 2011;**53**(11): 1120-1126. DOI: 10.1093/cid/cir627. Epub 2011 Oct 13

[46] Duffau P, Ozanne A, Bonnet F, Lazaro E, Cazanave C, Blanco P, et al. Multimorbidity, age-related comorbidities and mortality: Association of activation, senescence and inflammation markers in HIV adults. AIDS. 2018;**32**(12):1651-1660. DOI: 10.1097/QAD.0000000000001875

[47] Akinbami A, Bode-Shojobi I, Ajibola S, Oshinaike O, Adediran A, Ojelabi O, et al. Prevalence of asymptomatic bacteriuria in HIV infected patients in a tertiary Hospital in Lagos, Nigeria. World Journal of AIDS. 2013;**3**(2):105-110. DOI: 10.4236/wja.2013.32014

[48] Charanchi S, Kudi A, Tahir F. Antimicrobial sensitivity patterns of urogenital bacterial isolates among HIV positive patients in the Federal Medical Centre in Gombe. Internet Journal of Infectious Diseases. 2012;**10**(1):1-6

[49] Bent S, Nallamothu BK, Simel DL, Fihn SD, Saint S. Does this woman have an acute uncomplicated urinary tract infection? Journal of the American Medical Association. 2002;**287**(20): 2701-2710. DOI: 10.1001/jama.287.20.2701

[50] Fairley KF, Carson NE, Gutch RC, Leighton P, Grounds AD, Laird EC, et al. Site of infection in acute urinary-tract infection in general practice. Lancet. 1971;**2**(7725):615-618. DOI: 10.1016/s0140-6736(71)80066-1

[51] Millán-Rodríguez F, Palou J, Bujons-Tur A, Musquera-Felip M, Sevilla-Cecilia C, Serrallach-Orejas M, et al. Acute bacterial prostatitis: Two different sub-categories according to a previous manipulation of the lower urinary tract. World Journal of Urology. 2006;**24**(1): 45-50. DOI: 10.1007/s00345-005-0040-4.Epub 2005 Dec 31

[52] Nicolle LE. A practical guide to antimicrobial management of complicated urinary tract infection. Drugs & Aging. 2001;**18**(4):243-254. DOI: 10.2165/00002512-200118040-00002

[53] Bedi A, Miller CB, Hanson JL, Goodman S, Ambinder RF, Charache P, et al. Association of BK virus with failure of prophylaxis against hemorrhagic cystitis following bone marrow transplantation. Journal of Clinical Oncology. 1995;**13**(5):1103-1109. DOI: 10.1200/JCO.1995.13.5.1103

[54] Runde V, Ross S, Trenschel R, Lagemann E, Basu O, Renzing-Köhler K, et al. Adenoviral infection after allogeneic stem cell transplantation (SCT): Report on 130 patients from a single SCT unit involved in a prospective multi center surveillance study. Bone Marrow Transplantation. 2001;**28**(1): 51-57. DOI: 10.1038/sj.bmt.1703083

[55] Florescu MC, Miles CD, Florescu DF. What do we know about adenovirus in renal transplantation? Nephrology, Dialysis, Transplantation. 2013;**28**(8): 2003-2010. DOI: 10.1093/ndt/gft036. Epub 2013 Mar 13

[56] Drekonja DM, Rector TS, Cutting A, Johnson JR. Urinary tract infection in male veterans: Treatment patterns and outcomes. JAMA Internal Medicine. 2013;**173**(1):62-68. DOI: 10.1001/2013.jamainternmed.829

[57] Donlan RM. Biofilms and device-associated infections. Emerging Infectious Diseases. 2001;**7**(2):277-281. DOI: 10.3201/eid0702.010226

[58] Singha P, Locklin J, Handa H. A review of the recent advances in antimicrobial coatings for urinary catheters. Acta Biomaterialia. 2017;**50**: 20-40. DOI: 10.1016/j.actbio.2016.11.070. Epub 2016 Dec 1

[59] Al-Qas Hanna F, Sambirska O, Iyer S, Szpunar S, Fakih MG. Clinician practice and the National Healthcare Safety Network definition for the diagnosis of catheter-associated urinary tract infection. American Journal of Infection Control. 2013;**41**(12): 1173-1177. DOI: 10.1016/j.ajic.2013.05.024. Epub 2013 Sep 5

[60] Smithson A. Are health care-associated urinary tract infections properly defined? The American Journal of Emergency Medicine. 2011;**29**(4): 467-468; author reply 468-9. DOI: 10.1016/j.ajem.2010.12.034. Epub 2011 Feb 26

[61] Horan TC, Andrus M, Dudeck MA. CDC/NHSN surveillance definition of health care-associated infection and criteria for specific types of infections in the acute care setting. American Journal of Infection Control. 2008;**36**(5): 309-332. DOI: 10.1016/j.ajic.2008.03.002. Erratum in: American Journal of Infection Control 2008;**36**(9): 655

[62] Blodgett TJ, Gardner SE, Blodgett NP, Peterson LV, Pietraszak M. A tool to assess the signs and symptoms of catheter-associated urinary tract infection: Development and reliability. Clinical Nursing Research. 2015;**24**(4): 341-356. DOI: 10.1177/1054773814550506. Epub 2014 Sep 22

[63] Inouye SK, van Dyck CH, Alessi CA, Balkin S, Siegal AP, Horwitz RI. Clarifying confusion: The confusion assessment method. A new method for detection of delirium. Annals of Internal Medicine. 1990;**113**(12):941-948. DOI: 10.7326/0003-4819-113-12-941

[64] Vasilevskis EE, Morandi A, Boehm L, Pandharipande PP, Girard TD, Jackson JC, et al. Delirium and sedation recognition using validated instruments: Reliability of bedside intensive care unit nursing assessments from 2007 to 2010. Journal of the American Geriatrics Society. 2011;**59**(Suppl. 2):S249-S255. DOI: 10.1111/j.1532-5415.2011.03673.x

[65] Goetz AM, Squier C, Wagener MM, Muder RR. Nosocomial infections in the human immunodeficiency virus-infected patient: A two-year survey. American Journal of Infection Control. 1994;**22**(6):334-339. DOI: 10.1016/0196-6553(94)90031-0

[66] Padoveze MC, Trabasso P, Branchini ML. Nosocomial infections among HIV-positive and HIV-negative patients in a Brazilian infectious diseases unit. American Journal of Infection Control. 2002;**30**(6):346-350. DOI: 10.1067/mic.2002.125220

[67] The Centers for Disease Control and Prevention—CDC. Guideline for Prevention of Catheter-Associated Urinary Tract Infections (2009). HICPAC. Available from: https://www.cdc.gov/infectioncontrol/pdf/guidelines/cautiguidelines-H.pdf [Accessed: September 08, 2022]

[68] Krocová J, Prokešová R. Aspects of prevention of urinary tract infections associated with urinary bladder catheterisation and their implementation in nursing practice. Healthcare (Basel). 2022;**10**(1):152. DOI: 10.3390/healthcare10010152

[69] Gupta K, Hooton TM, Naber KG, Wullt B, Colgan R, Miller LG, et al. International clinical practice guidelines for the treatment of acute uncomplicated cystitis and pyelonephritis in women: A 2010 update by the Infectious Diseases Society of America and the European Society for Microbiology and Infectious Diseases. Clinical Infectious Diseases. 2011;**52**(5):e103-e120. DOI: 10.1093/cid/ciq257

[70] Kass EH. Bacteriuria and pyelonephritis of pregnancy. Archives of Internal Medicine. 1960;**105**:194-198. DOI: 10.1001/archinte.1960.00270140016003

[71] Norden CW, Kass EH. Bacteriuria of pregnancy—A critical appraisal. Annual Review of Medicine. 1968;**19**:431-470. DOI: 10.1146/annurev.me.19.020168.002243

[72] Warren JW, Tenney JH, Hoopes JM, Muncie HL, Anthony WC. A prospective microbiologic study of bacteriuria in patients with chronic indwelling urethral catheters. The Journal of Infectious Diseases. 1982;**146**(6):719-723. DOI: 10.1093/infdis/146.6.719

[73] Kincaid-Smith P, Bullen M. Bacteriuria in Pregnancy. Lancet. 1965; **1**(7382):395-399. DOI: 10.1016/s0140-6736(65)90001-2

[74] Bakke A, Digranes A. Bacteriuria in patients treated with clean intermittent catheterization. Scandinavian Journal of Infectious Diseases. 1991;**23**(5):577-582. DOI: 10.3109/00365549109105181

[75] Zhanel GG, Harding GK, Nicolle LE. Asymptomatic bacteriuria in patients with diabetes mellitus. Reviews of Infectious Diseases. 1991;**13**(1):150-154. DOI: 10.1093/clinids/12.5.150

[76] Nicolle LE, Bradley S, Colgan R, Rice JC, Schaeffer A, Hooton TM, et al. Infectious Diseases Society of America guidelines for the diagnosis and treatment of asymptomatic bacteriuria in adults. Clinical Infectious Diseases. 2005;**40**(5):643-654. DOI: 10.1086/427507. Epub 2005 Feb 4. Erratum in: Clinical Infectious Diseases 2005;**40**(10):1556

[77] Awolude OA, Adesina OA, Oladokun A, Mutiu WB, Adewole IF. Asymptomatic bacteriuria among HIV positive pregnant women. Virulence. 2010;**1**(3):130-133. DOI: 10.4161/viru.1.3.11384

[78] Widmer TA, Theron G, Grove D. Prevalence and risks of asymptomatic bacteriuria among HIV-positive pregnant women. Southern African Journal of Epidemiology and Infection. 2010;**25**(1):28-32. DOI: 10.1080/10158782.2010.11441374

[79] Ezechi OC, Gab-Okafor CV, Oladele DA, Kalejaiye OO, Oke BO, Ekama SO, et al. Prevalence and risk factors of asymptomatic bacteriuria among pregnant Nigerians infected with HIV. The Journal of Maternal-Fetal & Neonatal Medicine. 2013;**26**(4):402-406. DOI: 10.3109/14767058.2012.733782. Epub 2012 Nov 30

[80] Renuart AJ, Goldfarb DM, Mokomane M, Tawanana EO, Narasimhamurthy M, Steenhoff AP, et al. Microbiology of urinary tract infections in Gaborone, Botswana. PLoS One. 2013;**8**(3):e57776. DOI: 10.1371/journal.pone.0057776. Epub 2013 Mar 4

[81] Foxman B. The epidemiology of urinary tract infection. Nature Reviews. Urology. 2010;7(12):653-660. DOI: 10.1038/nrurol.2010.190

[82] Oli AN, Okafor CI, Ibezim EC, Akujiobi CN, Onwunzo MC. The prevalence and bacteriology of asymptomatic bacteriuria among antenatal patients in Nnamdi Azikiwe University Teaching Hospital Nnewi; South Eastern Nigeria. Nigerian Journal of Clinical Practice. 2010;**13**(4):409-412

[83] Vignesh R, Shankar EM, Murugavel KG, Kumarasamy N, Sekar R, Irene P, et al. Urinary infections due to multi-drug-resistant *Escherichia coli* among persons with HIV disease at a tertiary AIDS care centre in South India. Nephron. Clinical Practice. 2008;**110**(1): c55-c57. DOI: 10.1159/000151533

[84] Tessema NN, Ali MM, Zenebe MH. Bacterial associated urinary tract infection, risk factors, and drug susceptibility profile among adult people living with HIV at Haswassa University Comprehensive Specialized Hospital, Hawassa, Southern Esthiopia. Scientific Reports. 2020;**10**(1):10790. DOI: 10.1038/s41598-020-67840-7

[85] Skrzat-Klapaczyńska A, Matłosz B, Bednarska A, Paciorek M, Firląg-Burkacka E, Horban A, et al. Factors associated with urinary tract infections among HIV-1 infected patients. PLoS One. 2018;**13**(1):e0190564. DOI: 10.1371/journal.pone. 0190564

[86] Marami D, Balakrishnan S, Seyoum B. Prevalence, antimicrobial susceptibility pattern of bacterial isolates, and associated factors of urinary tract infections among HIV-positive patients at Hiwot Fana Specialized University Hospital, Eastern Ethiopia. Canadian Journal of Infectious Diseases and Medical Microbiology. 2019;**2019**: 6780354. DOI: 10.1155/2019/6780354

[87] Tchakoute CT, Liu J, Cohen B, Larson E. Risk factors and temporal trends of hospital-acquired infections (HAIs) among HIV positive patients in Urban New York City Hospitals: 2006 to 2014. Reviews on Recent Clinical Trials. 2017;**12**(1):44-50. DOI: 10.2174/1574887111666160906094140

[88] Sydnor ER, Perl TM. Hospital epidemiology and infection control in acute-care settings. Clinical Microbiology Reviews. 2011;**24**(1): 141-173. DOI: 10.1128/CMR.00027-10

[89] Park JC, Buono D, Smith DK, Peipert JF, Sobel J, Rompalo A, et al. Urinary tract infections in women with or at risk for human immunodeficiency virus infection. American Journal of Obstetrics and Gynecology. 2002;**187**(3): 581-588. DOI: 10.1067/mob.2002.125894

[90] Evans JK, McOwan A, Hillman RJ, Forster GE. Incidence of symptomatic urinary tract infections in HIV seropositive patients and the use of cotrimoxazole as prophylaxis against Pneumocystis carinii pneumonia. Genitourinary Medicine. 1995;**71**(2): 120-122. DOI: 10.1136/sti. 71.2.120

[91] Heyns CF, Fisher M. The urological management of the patient with acquired immunodeficiency syndrome. BJU International. 2005;**95**(5):709-716. DOI: 10.1111/j.1464-410X.2004.05435.x

[92] Mitchell TG, Perfect JR. Cryptococcosis in the era of AIDS—100 years after the discovery of *Cryptococcus neoformans*. Clinical Microbiology Reviews. 1995;**8**(4):515-548. DOI: 10.1128/CMR.8.4.515

[93] Wise GJ, Shteynshlyuger A. How to diagnose and treat fungal infections in

chronic prostatitis. Current Urology Reports. 2006;**7**(4):320-328. DOI: 10.1007/s11934-996-0012-2

[94] Marques LP, Rioja LS, Oliveira CA, Santos OD. AIDS-associated renal tuberculosis. Nephron. 1996;**74**(4): 701-704. DOI: 10.1159/000189477

[95] Van der Reijden HJ, Schipper ME, Danner SA, Arisz L. Glomerular lesions and opportunistic infections of the kidney in AIDS: An autopsy study of 47 cases. Advances in Experimental Medicine and Biology. 1989;**252**:181-188. DOI: 10.1007/978-1-4684-8953-8_18

[96] Dinnes J, Deeks J, Kunst H, Gibson A, Cummins E, Waugh N, et al. A systematic review of rapid diagnostic tests for the detection of tuberculosis infection. Health Technology Assessment. 2007;**11**(3):1-196. DOI: 10.3310/hta11030

[97] Moussa OM, Eraky I, El-Far MA, Osman HG, Ghoneim MA. Rapid diagnosis of genitourinary tuberculosis by polymerase chain reaction and non-radioactive DNA hybridization. The Journal of Urology. 2000;**164**(2):584-588

[98] Abubakar EM. Antimicrobial susceptibility pattern of pathogenic bacteria causing urinary tract infection at specialist hospital Yola Adamawa state Nigeria. Journal of Clinical Medical Research. 2009;**1**(1):001-008

[99] Wilson JM, Fenoff R. The Health and Economic Effects of Counterfeit Pharmaceuticals in Africa Anti-counterfeiting and Product Protection Program Backgrounder Series Global Edge Business Review 2011. Available from: http://royfenoff.com/Global_Edge_Business_Review_Article.pdf

[100] Bonkat G, Pickard R, Bartoletti R, et al. Guidelines on Urological Infections. Available from: https://uroweb.org/wp-content/uploads/EAU-Guidelines-on-Urological-Infections-2018-large-text.pdf [Accessed: February 2, 2022]

[101] Langner JL, Chiang KF, Stafford RS. Current prescribing practices and guideline concordance for the treatment of uncomplicated urinary tract infections in women. American Journal of Obstetrics and Gynecology. 2021;**225**(3): 272.e1-272.e11. DOI: 10.1016/j.ajog.2021.04.218. Epub 2021 Apr 20

[102] Cowart K, Worley M, Rouby NE, Sando K. Evaluation of FDA boxed warning on prescribing patterns of fluoroquinolones for uncomplicated urinary tract infections. The Annals of Pharmacotherapy. 2019;**53**(12): 1192-1199. DOI: 10.1177/1060028019865224. Epub 2019 Jul 18

[103] Lebovitch S, Mydlo JH. HIV-AIDS: Urologic considerations. The Urologic Clinics of North America. 2008;**35**(1): 59-68; vi. DOI: 10.1016/j.ucl.2007.09.001

[104] Adenis AA, Valdes A, Cropet C, McCotter OZ, Derado G, Couppie P, et al. Burden of HIV-associated histoplasmosis compared with tuberculosis in Latin America: A modelling study. The Lancet Infectious Diseases. 2018;**18**(10):1150-1159. DOI: 10.1016/S1473-3099(18)30354-2. Epub 2018 Aug 23

[105] Wall G, Lopez-Ribot JL. Current antimycotics, new prospects, and future approaches to antifungal therapy. Antibiotics (Basel). 2020;**9**(8):445. DOI: 10.3390/antibiotics 9080445

[106] Odabasi Z, Mert A. Candida urinary tract infections in adults. World Journal of Urology. 2020;**38**(11):2699-2707. DOI: 10.1007/s00345-019-02991-5. Epub 2019 Oct 25

[107] Cowen LE, Sanglard D, Howard SJ, Rogers PD, Perlin DS. Mechanisms of antifungal drug resistance. Cold Spring Harbor Perspectives in Medicine. 2014; **5**(7):a019752. DOI: 10.1101 /cshperspect. a019752

[108] Kauffman CA. Diagnosis and management of fungal urinary tract infection. Infectious Disease Clinics of North America. 2014;**28**(1):61-74. DOI: 10.1016/j.idc.2013.09.004. Epub 2013 Dec 8

[109] Pappas PG, Kauffman CA, Andes DR, Clancy CJ, Marr KA, Ostrosky-Zeichner L, et al. Clinical practice guideline for the Management of Candidiasis: 2016 update by the Infectious Diseases Society of America. Clinical Infectious Diseases. 2016;**62**(4): e1-e50. DOI: 10.1093/cid/civ933. Epub 2015 Dec 16

[110] Fisher JF, Sobel JD, Kauffman CA, Newman CA. Candida urinary tract infections—Treatment. Clinical Infectious Diseases. 2011;**52**(Suppl 6): S457-S466. DOI: 10.1093/cid/cir112

[111] Miceli MH, Kauffman CA. Isavuconazole: A new broad-spectrum triazole antifungal agent. Clinical Infectious Diseases. 2015;**61**(10): 1558-1565. DOI: 10.1093/cid/civ571. Epub 2015 Jul 15

[112] Felton T, Troke PF, Hope WW. Tissue penetration of antifungal agents. Clinical Microbiology Reviews. 2014; **27**(1):68-88. DOI: 10.1128/ CMR.00046-13

[113] Gabardi S, Martin S, Sura M, Mohammed A, Golan Y. Micafungin treatment and eradication of candiduria among hospitalized patients. International Urology and Nephrology. 2016;**48**(11):1881-1885. DOI: 10.1007/ s11255-016-1410-0. Epub 2016 Sep 1

[114] Grau S, Luque S, Echeverría-Esnal D, Sorlí L, Campillo N, Montero M, et al. Urinary micafungin levels are sufficient to treat urinary tract infections caused by Candida spp. International Journal of Antimicrobial Agents. 2016;**48**(2): 212-214. DOI: 10.1016/j.ijantimicag. 2016.05.010. Epub 2016 Jul 5

[115] Sobel JD, Bradshaw SK, Lipka CJ, Kartsonis NA. Caspofungin in the treatment of symptomatic candiduria. Clinical Infectious Diseases. 2007;**44**(5): e46-e49. DOI: 10.1086/510432. Epub 2007 Jan 22

[116] Chen SC, Slavin MA, Sorrell TC. Echinocandin antifungal drugs in fungal infections: A comparison. Drugs. 2011; **71**(1):11-41. DOI: 10.2165/ 11585270-000000000-00000 Erratum in: Drugs 2011;**71**(2):253

[117] Sucher AJ, Chahine EB, Balcer HE. Echinocandins: The newest class of antifungals. The Annals of Pharmacotherapy. 2009;**43**(10): 1647-1657. DOI: 10.1345/aph.1M237. Epub 2009 Sep 1

[118] Janknegt R, de Marie S, Bakker-Woudenberg IA, Crommelin DJ. Liposomal and lipid formulations of amphotericin B. Clinical Pharmacokinetics. 1992;**23**(4):279-291. DOI: 10.2165/00003088-199223040-00004

[119] Hakki M. Moving past ganciclovir and Foscarnet: Advances in CMV therapy. Current Hematologic Malignancy Reports. 2020;**15**(2):90-102. DOI: 10.1007/s11899-020-00557-6

[120] Nahid P, Dorman SE, Alipanah N, Barry PM, Brozek JL, Cattamanchi A, et al. Executive summary: Official American Thoracic Society/Centers for Disease Control and Prevention/ Infectious Diseases Society of America

Clinical Practice Guidelines: Treatment of drug-susceptible tuberculosis. Clinical Infectious Diseases. 2016;**63**(7):853-867. DOI: 10.1093/cid/ciw566

[121] Snider DE Jr. Pyridoxine supplementation during isoniazid therapy. Tubercle. 1980;**61**(4):191-196. DOI: 10.1016/0041-3879(80)90038-0

[122] Visser ME, Texeira-Swiegelaar C, Maartens G. The short-term effects of anti-tuberculosis therapy on plasma pyridoxine levels in patients with pulmonary tuberculosis. The International Journal of Tuberculosis and Lung Disease. 2004;**8**(2):260-262

[123] Benator D, Bhattacharya M, Bozeman L, Burman W, Cantazaro A, Chaisson R, et al. Rifapentine and isoniazid once a week versus rifampicin and isoniazid twice a week for treatment of drug-susceptible pulmonary tuberculosis in HIV-negative patients: A randomised clinical trial. Lancet. 2002; **360**(9332):528-534. DOI: 10.1016/s0140-6736(02)09742-8

[124] Vernon A, Burman W, Benator D, Khan A, Bozeman L. Acquired rifamycin monoresistance in patients with HIV-related tuberculosis treated with once-weekly rifapentine and isoniazid. Tuberculosis Trials Consortium. Lancet. 1999;**353**(9167):1843-1847. DOI: 10.1016/s0140-6736(98)11467-8

[125] Burman W, Benator D, Vernon A, Khan A, Jones B, Silva C, et al. Acquired rifamycin resistance with twice-weekly treatment of HIV-related tuberculosis. American Journal of Respiratory and Critical Care Medicine. 2006;**173**(3): 350-356. DOI: 10.1164/rccm.200503-417OC. Epub 2005 Aug 18

[126] Abdool Karim SS, Naidoo K, Grobler A, Padayatchi N, Baxter C, Gray A, et al. Timing of initiation of antiretroviral drugs during tuberculosis therapy. The New England Journal of Medicine. 2010;**362**(8):697-706. DOI: 10.1056/NEJMoa0905848

[127] Justesen US, Andersen AB, Klitgaard NA, Brøsen K, Gerstoft J, Pedersen C. Pharmacokinetic interaction between rifampin and the combination of indinavir and low-dose ritonavir in HIV-infected patients. Clinical Infectious Diseases. 2004;**38**(3):426-429. DOI: 10.1086/380794. Epub 2004 Jan 12

[128] Ueaphongsukkit T, Gatechompol S, Sophonphan J, et al. Efficacy and PK of dolutegravir 50 mg QD with food versus 50 mg BID with rifampicin. Virtual Conference on Retroviruses and Opportunistic Infections. 2021. Abstract 370

[129] Luetkemeyer AF, Kendall MA, Nyirenda M, Wu X, Ive P, Benson CA, et al. Tuberculosis immune reconstitution inflammatory syndrome in A5221 STRIDE: Timing, severity, and implications for HIV-TB programs. Journal of Acquired Immune Deficiency Syndromes. 2014;**65**(4):423-428. DOI: 10.1097/QAI.0000000000000030

[130] Meintjes G, Lawn SD, Scano F, Maartens G, French MA, Worodria W, et al. International network for the study of HIV-associated IRIS. Tuberculosis-associated immune reconstitution inflammatory syndrome: Case definitions for use in resource-limited settings. The Lancet Infectious Diseases. 2008;**8**(8):516-523. DOI: 10.1016/S1473-3099(08)70184-1

[131] Meintjes G, Wilkinson RJ, Morroni C, Pepper DJ, Rebe K, Rangaka MX, et al. Randomized placebo-controlled trial of prednisone for paradoxical tuberculosis-associated immune reconstitution inflammatory syndrome. AIDS. 2010;**24**(15): 2381-2390. DOI: 10.1097/QAD.0b013e32833dfc68

Chapter 4

Emphysematous Urinary Tract Infections

Guadalupe Aguirre Avalos

Abstract

Emphysematous urinary tract infections are severe necrotizing infections of the urinary tract. The descriptive term emphysematous is used for the gas location site: pyelonephritis, pyelitis, and cystitis. Most cases occur in adult females. Diabetes mellitus constitutes the most commonly associated comorbidity and a risk factor for necrotizing infections. Pathogenesis still needs to be fully understood. *Escherichia coli* is the most common microorganism, followed by *Klebsiella pneumonia, Proteus mirabilis*, and *Pseudomonas aeruginosa.* Bacteremia occurs in more than half of cases. The treatment includes resuscitation, glycemic control, and antimicrobial therapy, followed by early drainage. Emphysematous cystitis is the most common and frequently least morbid gas-forming urinary tract infection. Using minimally invasive image-guided procedures for drainage of gas and abscess is a conservative strategy with renal preservation, while emergency nephrectomy is considered the last option. Mortality rates have a direct correlation between the computed tomography findings and the modalities of treatment.

Keywords: necrotizing urinary tract infection, emphysematous urinary tract infections, emphysematous pyelonephritis, emphysematous pyelitis, emphysematous cystitis

1. Introduction

Emphysematous urinary tract infections are severe necrotizing infections characterized by the presence of gas. Classification is based on the gas location site and extent: emphysematous pyelonephritis is gas in the renal parenchyma and the surrounding tissues; emphysematous pyelitis is gas only in the collecting system; emphysematous cystitis is gas within the bladder wall and lumen. The coexistence of emphysematous pyelonephritis (EPN) and emphysematous cystitis (EC) is uncommon. The cases of pneumaturia in which gas develops in the urinary tract through some fermenting microorganism were described in 1898 [1]. Other researchers have confirmed that the mixed acid fermentation of glucose by microorganisms is the primary pathway of gas formation [2]. The term emphysematous pyelonephritis was first used in 1962, with the first series of cases included from 1989 to 1962 [3]. The diagnostic challenge in these infections is that clinical manifestations do not distinguish the severity of necrotizing infections. The diagnosis depends on detecting gas in or around the kidney, collecting system, or bladder. The best diagnostic method is computed tomography (CT) to confirm EPN [4]. Empiric antimicrobial therapy should primarily target *Escherichia coli*, *Klebsiella pneumoniae*, *Proteus mirabilis*, and *Pseudomonas aeruginosa*. The current trend in using minimally invasive procedures for EPN is to perform a percutaneous intervention or internal drainage in most patients [5]. The case series EPN from 1980 to 2011 showed a mortality rate of 18% [4].

2. Emphysematous pyelonephritis

EPN is a severe necrotizing infection characterized by gas in the renal parenchyma and the surrounding tissues. The term EPN was first used in 1962 with a report of a female with a tender mass in the right flank. Her abdomen X-ray revealed gas surrounding and infiltrating the right kidney. Retrograde pyelogram showed that renal calyces and pelvis are compressed and displaced medially by a gaseous inflammatory process [3].

2.1 Epidemiology

Most reported cases of EPN occur in adult patients. The incidence is higher in females than males, with a preponderance (3:1) and mean age of 56.6 years. Diabetes mellitus (DM) constituted the most commonly associated comorbidity and a risk factor for EPN, with an incidence of 85% [4, 6, 7]. Other comorbidities include urolithiasis, a previous history of treated pyelonephritis, and chronic kidney disease [6]. To date, few cases of EPN have been reported in pediatric patients. Risk factors for pediatric: neurogenic bladder, ureteropelvic junction obstruction, obstruction due to ectopic ureter, renal stone, nephro-urological congenital malformation, congenital ureterocele, and acquired immunodeficiency [8]. The left kidney is most commonly affected in 52–67%, on the right side in 25–37.7%, and bilateral in 10.2–15.3% [4, 6, 7, 9].

2.2 Pathogenesis

The pathogenesis of EPN is not yet fully understood; it could be different between patients with diabetes and no diabetics. The cases of pneumaturia in which gas develops in the urinary tract through some fermenting microorganisms were described in 1898 [1]. Mixed acid fermentation of glucose by microorganisms is the primary pathway of gas formation. Emphysematous infection in the urinary tract requires four critical conditions to develop: (1) the presence of gas-forming bacteria or fungi, (2) high local tissue glucose level, (3) impaired tissue perfusion, and (4) an inadequate immune response [2].

A urinary tract obstruction is seen in 75% of patients. It is attributable to ureteric calculi, renal papillary necrosis, ureteric stricture, and fungal bezoar [7]. Urolithiasis may be the most important contributing factor in the pathogenesis of EPN among no patients with diabetes [5]. Accumulating the gas in unrelieved urinary tract obstruction can raise pelvicalyceal pressure. Further impairing renal circulation results in poor tissue perfusion and infective parenchymal destruction [7].

A gross examination of nephrectomy specimens shows multiple abscesses in the renal parenchyma. On microscopic examination: blurred corticomedullary differentiation, congested medulla, patchy areas of hemorrhage, empty spaces, acute inflammatory cell infiltration in the surrounding areas, vasculitis, extensive necrosis, microscopic abscesses, glomerulosclerosis, arteriosclerosis, intrarenal vascular thrombi, and infarcts, or papillary necrosis [10–12].

2.3 Clinical presentation

The clinical manifestation and urinalysis do not distinguish the different types and severity of pyelonephritis. In EPN, the mean duration from the onset of symptoms to diagnosis ranged from 4 to 11 days [12]. Clinical manifestations of EPN include fever and rigors in 74.7%, flank pain in 70.4%, acute renal failure in 45.2–80%, pneumaturia in 35%, and shock in 24.6%. Septic shock at admission indicates a poor prognosis. A palpable tender kidney has been identified as one of the poor clinical prognostic parameters requiring prompt intervention and intensive monitoring. Approximately 40.4% of the patients require admission to the intensive care unit [4, 6, 11, 13].

2.4 Diagnosis

Laboratory findings demonstrate leukocytosis in 70.9% and thrombocytopenia in 25.8% [14]. Urinalysis results are positive for pyuria and hematuria [4, 7, 15]. Urine culture identified *E. coli* as the most common infective microorganism, followed by *K. pneumoniae, Proteus* sp., *Pseudomonas* sp., *Candida albicans, and Enterococcus* sp., among others [4–6, 9, 15, 16]. Polymicrobial infections are found in 10–23.5% [10, 16]. Extended-spectrum β–lactamase-producing Gram-negative pathogens are found in 39% of the cases [7]. Bacteremia occurs in more than half of cases (54–75%). The blood culture is positive for the same microorganism identified in the urine. *E. coli* and *K. pneumoniae* are the most common microorganisms in blood cultures [4, 6, 9, 10].

The diagnosis depends on detecting gas in or around the kidney. The best diagnostic method is CT to confirm EPN, which also aids in staging the EPN and underlying urinary tract obstruction. While the accuracy rate for ultrasonography is 67.9% and for X-ray film of the abdomen is 53.2% [4, 7].

Classification of EPN is based on radiological imaging. The most commonly used is the CT scan classification system Huang-Tseng. This classification established the location and extent of gas or abscess in the renal parenchyma and surrounding tissues. The classification focused on the radiological severity, prognosis, and management: class 1, gas in the collecting system; class 2, gas in the renal parenchyma without extension to extrarenal space; class 3A, an extension of gas or abscess to perinephric space; class 3B, an extension of gas or abscess to pararenal space; and class 4, bilateral involvement or solitary kidney with EPN [9].

2.5 Treatment

There are different treatment options and effective ways of initial management of EPN, which improves survival and helps preserve renal function. Employing different measures, which include aggressive resuscitation, glycemic control, and parenteral antimicrobial therapy followed by early drainage of the infected fluid, as well as gas and release of urinary tract obstruction [7].

2.5.1 Antimicrobial therapy

Empiric antimicrobial therapy should primarily target *E. coli*, *K. pneumoniae*, *P. mirabilis*, *P. aeruginosa*, and *Enterococcus* sp. Third-generation cephalosporins are recommended as initial treatment. Carbapenems are the empiric therapy of choice in patients, with histories of prior hospitalization, antibiotic use, those needing emergency hemodialysis or developing disseminated intravascular coagulation, and clinically unstable patients irrespective of CT findings (low/high risk) [16, 17]. There has yet to be a consensus on the duration of antimicrobial therapy for ENP. At the time of discharge, the duration of treatment could reach ≥4 weeks [18].

2.5.2 Minimally invasive procedures

Using minimally invasive image-guided procedures for drainage of the gas and abscess is a conservative strategy with renal preservation. In 1986, EPN was successful management by percutaneous drainage (PCD) under fluoroscopic guidance and medical management [19]. This report was followed by CT-guided interventional drainage. PCD tube placement is best done with CT guidance. Monitoring response to PCD, CT was done 4 to 7 days later to ascertain the location of the catheter and assess the abscess resolution. Catheters were removed when follow-up scans indicated complete resolution. Antimicrobial therapy with PCD was associated with improved survival rates [20]. The PCD and relief of urinary tract obstruction (if it exists) combined with antimicrobial therapy is the choice for class 1 or 2 of the CT scan classification system Huang-Tseng. However, for extensive classes, 3 or 4 may be attempted too [9].

Other alternative intervention strategies include JJ stent insertion or percutaneous nephrostomy insertion. [6] The preference for placing JJ stents as the choice of drainage procedure is because it can be performed endoscopically [15]. The current trend in using minimally invasive procedures for EPN is to perform a percutaneous intervention or internal drainage in most patients [5].

2.5.3 Open surgical drainage

Available evidence has suggested that if antimicrobial therapy with PCD is not improving the patient's condition, open surgical drainage must be considered before considering a nephrectomy [4]. Perinephric and extensive pararenal abscesses are other indications for open surgical drainage with the placement of large caliber tubes. Opening the Gerota fascia in cases of perinephric collections is a crucial and rewarding step to drain the gas and infected fluid [7].

2.5.4 Emergency nephrectomy

Since the early series reported, the immediate nephrectomy has been a subject of controversy [10, 12]. More recently, kidney preservation should be the primary goal in treating EPN when the differential renal clearance is >10% because the preserved kidneys maintained their function during the follow-up [13, 17]. Emergency nephrectomy is considered the last option. Furthermore, it is reserved only for patients with extensive EPN and fulminant courses or for patients who can not be stabilized despite aggressive resuscitation or by failure percutaneous measures. [5, 7, 9] Considering these indications, the number of patients requiring emergency nephrectomy is 6% [5–7, 17].

2.6 Mortality

Mortality rates had a direct correlation with the CT findings and the modalities of treatment. Patients with extensive EPN class 3B or 4 of the CT scan-classification system Huang-Tsengn had a high mortality rate of 45% [11]. The mortality rate approached 46% among patients who received medical treatment only [12]. Using minimally invasive procedures with medical treatment showed a mortality rate of 18.8% [4, 5]. Risk stratification of the lethality of the EPN based on the prognostic scoring system reaches an overall mortality rate of <6%. A score of 1–8 is very low risk, a score of 9–15 is low-risk, a score of 16–20 is intermediate risk, and a score of >20 is high risk. A higher prognostic score was associated with mortality. Identifying prognostic indicators and risk stratification allow prompt and appropriate medical and surgical treatments [6].

The factors associated with mortality: systolic BP <90 mm Hg at admission, decreased platelet count <100,000/mm^3, urine culture for *E. coli*, hyponatremia, radiological severity with higher CT grade at admission, higher creatinine levels, and emergency nephrectomy [5, 14]. Over 54% of patients with septic shock died from EPN [4]. Early risk stratification, intensive management, and prompt treatment according to a protocol can reduce mortality even further in patients with EPN [17].

3. Emphysematous pyelitis

Emphysematous pyelitis (gas only in the collecting system-class1) is classified into mild class EPN with a better prognosis. In this class, conservative management should be considered [4].

4. Coexistence of emphysematous pyelonephritis and emphysematous cystitis

The coexistence is an uncommon presentation that has been reported rarely [11]. Patients with EC can progress ascending emphysematous infections, and 10.2% may subsequently develop EPN, which could significantly increase the associated morbidity and mortality of these infections [21–23].

5. Emphysematous cystitis

Emphysematous cystitis (gas within the bladder wall and lumen) is the most common and frequently the least morbid gas-forming urinary tract infection.

5.1 Epidemiology

The incidence of EC is unknown since the number of EC might be underdiagnosed, as imaging studies are not routinely used in patients with urinary tract infections. The main risk factors for EC are DM in 70%, chronic kidney disease, neurogenic bladder, recurrent urinary tract infection, and urinary stasis secondary to bladder outlet obstruction [21, 23].

5.2 Anatomopathological findings

A pathological assessment of involved bladder tissue might show bladder wall thickening with vesicles of varying size. Microscopic findings showed multiple gas-filled vesicles predominantly within the bladder mucosa lined by flattened fibrocytes and multinucleated giant cells [24].

5.3 Clinical presentation

Patients can be asymptomatic in 7%, with diagnosis incidental to abdominal imaging for other concurrent illnesses [23]. Symptoms of acute cystitis are nonspecific and usually mild; dysuria, urinary frequency, and urinary urgency occur in approximately 50% of patients. Fever may be observed in approximately 30–50%. Other symptoms may be present, such as abdominal pain and hematuria [22].

5.4 Diagnosis

E. coli is the most common cause of EC in 40.4%, followed by *Klebsiella pneumonia*, *Enterobacter aerogenes*, *P. mirabilis*, and *Streptococcus* spp. Extended-spectrum β–lactamase-producing Gram-negative pathogens are identified in 36.5% [21]. EC is diagnosed by: radiological studies, through direct visualization on cystoscopy, and during laparotomy, on tissue from bladder biopsy or autopsy. Most cases are diagnosed using simple plain films of the abdomen, 84%. CT detects cases of EC that are not apparent on plain abdominal films. CT accurately defines the extent and severity of EC and allows an assessment of ascending infection [23].

5.5 Treatment

Most patients are treated successfully with glycemic control, antimicrobial treatment, urethral catheterization, and hydration [21, 23]. The severity of the EC determines the surgical method. Surgical involved cystectomy, partial cystectomy, or debridement. Surgery is required in patients exhibiting a poor response to initial medical management or those with severe necrotizing infection.

5.6 Mortality

The overall death rate of EC is 7%. Among the patients that die are the following associated conditions: septic shock, late presentation, perforation of the bladder, and nonresponse to medical therapy [22, 23].

6. Case report

A 51-year-old man was admitted to the hospital with malaise, left flank pain, fever, chills, and dysuria lasting 5 days. He has a history of 20 years with diabetes mellitus and hypertension, receiving insulin, metformin, and telmisartan therapy. On physical examination, he had a 103/52 mm Hg blood pressure with mild left costovertebral angle tenderness. Laboratory values revealed impaired renal function with a serum creatinine of 3.2 mg/dL and blood urea of 198.5 mg/dL. Procalcitonin of 12.9 ng/ml, white blood cell counts of 19×10^9/L, HbA1c 9.7%, D-dimer of 1707 ng/ml, and glycosuria. An urgent abdominal CT scan showed class 3B, CT scan-classification system Huang-Tseng with an extension of gas or abscess to pararenal space (**Figure 1**) and EC. Initial empiric antimicrobial therapy with ertapenem started. On day 1 of admission, the patient was transferred to the intensive care unit after open surgical drainage of gas, an abscess of 80 mL, and placement of large caliber tubes. At the time of admission, he was intubated with a blood pressure of 95/51 mm Hg and vasopressor support. The sequential organ failure assessment (SOFA) score was 8, with an estimated

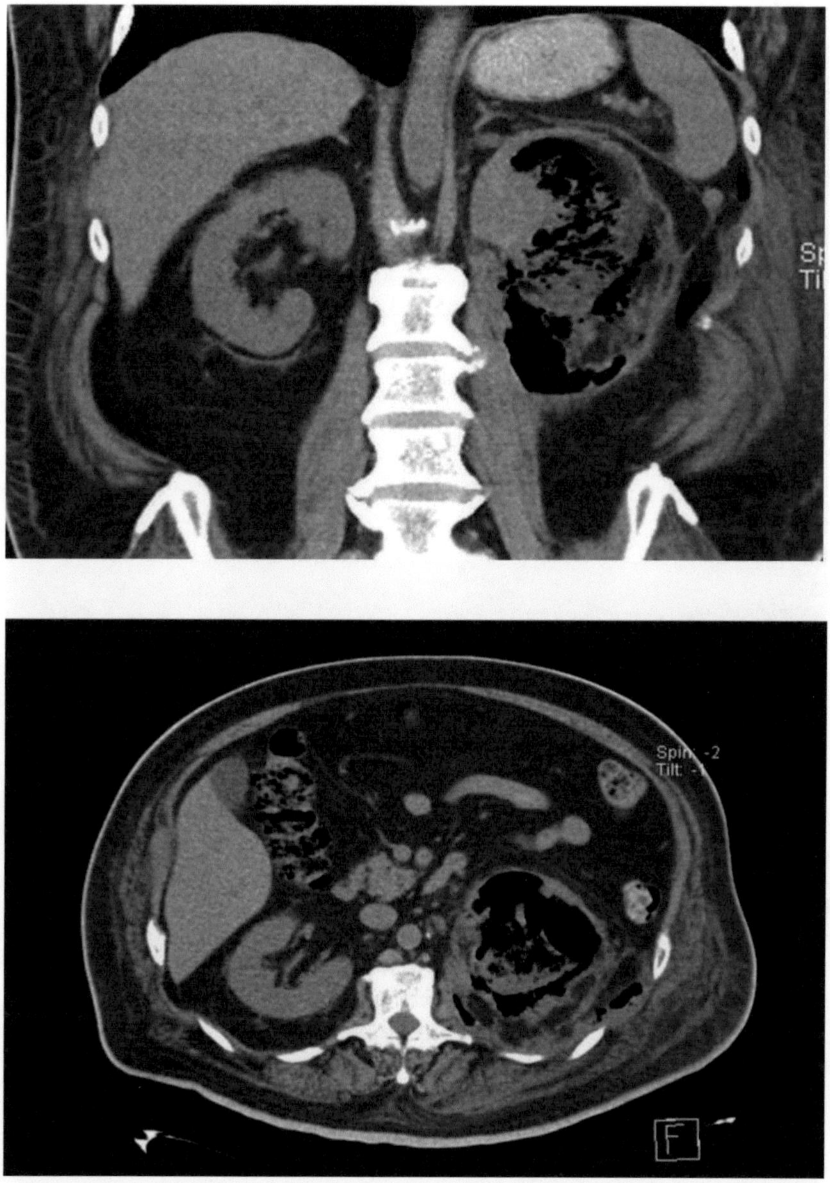

Figure 1.
CT scan of a 51-year-old male with left side class 3B ENP CT scan-classification system Huang-Tseng with an extension of gas and abscess to pararenal space. It shows an enlarged left kidney with intraparenchymal gas.

mortality of 15–20%. SOFA score was used to quantify the degree of organ dysfunction or failure present on admission and stratify for mortality prediction in intensive care unit patients. The acute physiology and chronic health disease classification system (APACHE) II score was 22, with an estimated mortality of 57.4%. This score includes weightage for age, past comorbid conditions, acute physiological parameters, emergency surgery, and reason for intensive care unit admission. APACHE II score was designed to measure the severity of disease for adult patients admitted to intensive care units. After 4 days in the intensive care unit, he was transferred back to the ward. On day 22 of hospitalization, open surgical drainage of an abscess in a pararenal space

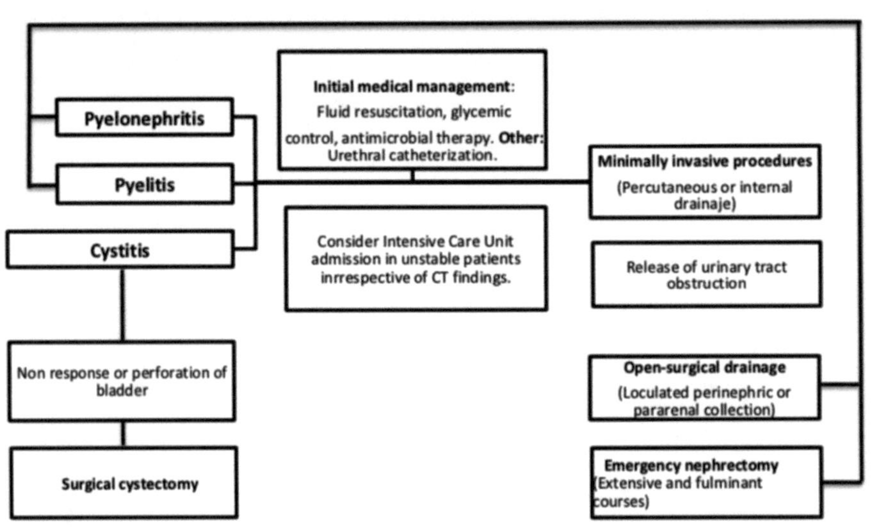

Figure 2.
Management of emphysematous urinary tract infections.

of 200 mL with debridement was realized. On day 27, a nephrectomy was performed (**Figure 2**). *E. coli* was isolated from urine and abscess with the same sensitivity pattern and positive for extended-spectrum β–lactamase. He received meropenem for 4 weeks, and his renal function gradually returned to normal. He was discharged after 44 days of hospital stay.

7. Conclusions

Emphysematous urinary tract infections are severe necrotizing infections of the urinary tract. Septic shock at admission and a palpable tender kidney have been identified as poor clinical prognostic parameters. The diagnosis depends on detecting gas in or around the urinary tract. The best diagnostic method is CT to confirm emphysematous urinary tract infections. Extended-spectrum β–lactamase-producing Gram-negative pathogens are found in high percentages of cases. This type of resistance is a global public health concern. Mortality rates had a direct correlation with the CT findings and the modalities of treatment.

Acknowledgements

We thank Amaya-Aguirre KI and Leyva-Villarreal DM for assisting in the preparation of the manuscript. A special thanks to Gómez-Partida CA, Hernández-Lugo D, Gamero-Rodríguez MJ, Ochoa-Saaib J, Ayala-Delgadillo NT, Angeles-Uribe JM, Jiménez-Pérez DM, and all ICU health care staff for their support in-patient care.

Author details

Guadalupe Aguirre Avalos
Universidad de Guadalajara, Centro Universitario de Ciencias de la Salud,
Guadalajara Jalisco, México

*Address all correspondence to: gaguirre.investigacion@gmail.com

References

[1] Kelly HA, MacCallum WG. Pneumaturia. The Journal of the American Medical Association. 1898;**XXXI**(8):375-381

[2] Huang JJ, Chen KW, Ruaan MK. Mixed acid fermentation of glucose as a mechanism of emphysematous urinary tract infection. The Journal of Urology. 1991;**146**(1):148-151

[3] Schultz EH, Klorfein EH. Emphysematous pyelonephritis. Journal of Urology. 1962;**87**(6):762-766

[4] Aboumarzouk OM et al. Emphysematous pyelonephritis: Time for a management plan with an evidence-based approach. Arab Journal of Urology. 2014;**12**(2):106-115

[5] Kamath SU, Patil B, Shelke U, Patwardhan SK. Comparing diabetic and nondiabetic emphysematous pyelonephritis and evaluating predictors of mortality. Saudi Journal of Kidney Diseases and Transplantation. 2019;**30**(6):1266-1275

[6] Krishnamoorthy S, Zumla A, Sekar H, Muneer A, Thiruvengadam G, Kumaresan N. Prognostic scoring system and risk stratification in patients with emphysematous pyelonephritis: An 11-year prospective study at a tertiary referral centre. BJU International. 2020;**127**(4):418-427

[7] Adapala RR, Shetty R, Venugopal P, Prabhu GGL, Yalla D, Unnikrishnan B. Renal salvage, an achievable goal in patients with emphysematous pyelonephritis: Outcomes of an algorithmic renal preserving strategy. Urology Annals. 2020;**12**(2):156-162

[8] Kitano H et al. Case report: Emphysematous pyelonephritis with a congenital giant ureterocele. Frontiers in Pediatrics. 2021;**9**:1-5

[9] Huang JJ, Tseng CC. Emphysematous pyelonephritis: Clinicoradiological classification, management, prognosis, and pathogenesis. Archives of Internal Medicine. 2002;**160**(6):797-805

[10] Shokeir AA, El-Azab M, Mohsen T, El-Diasty T. Emphysematous pyelonephritis: A 15-Year Experience with 20 cases. Urology. 1997;**49**:343-346

[11] Dutta P et al. Presentation and outcome of emphysematous renal tract disease in patients with diabetes mellitus. Urologia Internationalis. 2007;**78**(1):13-22

[12] Wan YL, Lee TY, Bullard MJ, Tsai CC. Acute gas-producing bacterial renal infection: Correlation between imaging findings and clinical outcome. Radiology. 1996;**198**(2):433-438

[13] El-Nahas AR et al. Kidney preservation protocol for management of emphysematous pyelonephritis: Treatment modalities and follow-up. Arab Journal of Urology. 2011;**9**(3):185-189

[14] Olvera-Posada D et al. Emphysematous pyelonephritis: Multicenter clinical and therapeutic experience in Mexico. Urology. 2014;**83**(6):1280-1284

[15] Das D, Pal DK. Double J stenting: A rewarding option in the management of emphysematous pyelonephritis. Urology Annals. 2016;**8**(3):261-264

[16] Lu YC et al. Recommended initial antimicrobial therapy for emphysematous pyelonephritis. Medicine (Baltimore). 2016;**95**(21):1-7

[17] Kone K, Mallikarjun NT, Keerthi Rams MDRK. Mortality in emphysematous pyelonephritis. Can we reduce it further by using a protocol-based treatment? The results of a prospective study. Urology Annals. 2022;**14**(1):73-80

[18] Kapoor R et al. Predictive factors for mortality and need for nephrectomy in patients with emphysematous pyelonephritis. BJU International. 2010;**105**(7):986-989

[19] Hudson MA, Weyman PJ, Van Der Vliet AH, Catalona WJ. Emphysematous pyelonephritis: Successful management by percutaneous drainage. The Journal of Urology. 1986;**136**(4):884-886

[20] Chen MT, Huang CN, Chou YH, Huang CH, Chiang CP, Liu GC. Percutaneous drainage in the treatment of emphysematous pyelonephritis: 10-Year experience. The Journal of Urology. 1997;**157**(5):1569-1573

[21] Choi J, Choi SK, Lee SH, Yoo KH. Clinical outcomes and risk factor analysis of patients presenting with emphysematous cystitis: A 15-year retrospective multicenter study. Medicina (B. Aires). 2021;**57**(531):1-7

[22] Amano M, Shimizu T. Emphysematous cystitis: A review of the literature. Internal Medicine. 2014;**53**(2):79-82

[23] Thomas AA, Lane BR, Thomas AZ, Remer EM, Campbell SC, Shoskes DA. Emphysematous cystitis: A review of 135 cases. BJU International. 2007;**100**(1):17-20

[24] Rocca JM, McClure J. Cystitis Emphysematosa. Britsh Journal of Urology. 1985;**57**(5):585

Section 3

Diagnosis of Urinary Tract Infections

Chapter 5

Noninvasive Bladder Volume Monitoring Using Bioimpedance

Víctor Hugo Mosquera

Abstract

Due to the electrical conductivity of the urine, several bioimpedance techniques have been considered for bladder volume monitoring. This chapter shows several approaches for bladder volume estimation; among these, Global Impedance (GI), presents a high accuracy in volume estimation. Other proposed approaches are Voltage Change Ratios (VCR), Impedance Ratio Method (IRM), and Focused Impedance Method (FIM), which presents highly sensitive to changes in the conductivity, just like GI. Therefore, these approaches are not suitable for long-term monitoring of the bladder, because the conductivity of urine varies with health status and diet. The proposal FIM-IE presents a low sensibility to the conductivity uncertainty; being a promising technique for long-term monitoring of the bladder and would support the assisted bladder emptying process.

Keywords: bioimpedance, bladder volume monitoring, EIT, global impedance, impedance ratio, voltage change ratio

1. Introduction

Electrical impedance tomography (EIT) is a noninvasive technique to obtain images of the internal conductivity of an object. The EIT systems are based on the injection of current signals and the measurement of the generated potentials at the boundary of the object under study. In EIT applications on biological tissues, the currents are usually sinusoidal, with amplitudes below 1 mA and frequencies ranging from 1 kHz to 100 kHz. Once the potentials and currents are known, an image reconstruction method is used to estimate the spatial distribution of the internal electrical conductivity of the analyzed object [1].

The so-called vesicoureteral reflux is a pathology that is presented by the leakage of urine from the bladder to the kidneys. This pathology can generate chronic renal failure, urinary tract and kidney infections, nephrotic syndrome, and scarring of the kidneys, among others. For this reason, the EIT seeks to monitor the bladder volume and support the diagnosis of this pathology [2]. It is the case of Li and colleagues [3], who designed an EIT system based on 16 electrodes, with a frequency range from 0 to 12.5 MHz; this system monitors the distribution of impedance in the bladder, and so establishes a close relationship between the bladder volume and estimated conductivity in healthy patients. On the other hand, Schlebusch and collaborators [4–6], with the aim of assist to paraplegic patients, which present decreased bladder volume sensation due to damage to their neuronal structures, and used the EIT to monitor the bladder volume.

This chapter presents several bioimpedance indexes for bladder size monitoring, such as Global Impedance (GI), Voltage Change Ratio (VCR), and Impedance Ratio Method (IRM), which show promising results in bladder volume estimation, with the limitation that they are highly sensitive to urine conductivity. On the other hand, methods based on Focused Impedance Measurement (FIM) are presented, which have a matrix electrode configuration, different from the classical ring arrangement of the GI, VCR, and IRM methods; this matrix arrangement allows for decreasing the sensitivity of urine conductivity in the process of bladder volume estimation.

2. Urodynamics

The study of lower urinary tract function is called urodynamics, which consists of monitoring the filling and emptying of the bladder for the diagnosis and management of lower urinary tract dysfunction. This dysfunction occurs in elderly people or those with neural disorders, such as spinal cord diseases, which generate urinary incontinence (UI), detrusor hyperactivity, and prostatic hyperplasia, pathologies that cause urinary tract infections [7, 8].

Urodynamics is currently performed by means of filling cytometry, pressure-flow studies, uroflowmetry, and electromyography [9]. Cystometry is an invasive ambulatory technique that is performed by medical professionals in a Urology Unit. For this technique, a small amount of liquid at room temperature is injected through a catheter and then another equal amount of warm liquid; the patient indicates when the sensation of urination begins; when the bladder is full the patient proceeds to empty the bladder; finally, the catheter is removed from the urinary tract. During this procedure, the pressure in the bladder is measured by a cytometer [8, 10]. On the other hand, the pressure-flow study allows analysis of bladder and detrusor pressure; to determine urinary tract obstructions and alterations in detrusor contraction. This technique involves the use of a probe inside the patient's urethra to measure the detrusor pressure, so it must be performed by trained personnel [10]. Electromyography is an electrophysiological test that measures muscle activity simultaneously with cystometry. This technique seeks to detect striated muscle activity and evaluates nerve integrity, location, and severity of the lesion [10].

Another method is uroflowmetry, which measures external urine flow per unit time (Q ml/s). This is a noninvasive technique for measuring urinary flow. The patient voids the bladder into a flowmeter when he/she has the sensation of urination. This measurement reflects the kinetics of detrusor contraction. This method cannot be used as the only alternative for the diagnosis of urinary tract pathologies [7, 8, 10].

Invasive methods of urodynamic studies can cause irritation of the urethra or bladder from catheter insertion, urethral bleeding or bloody urination, infection through the catheter, urethral fistula at catheter placement, and bladder wall rupture at catheter placement [10].

EIT is a noninvasive, radiation-free clinical monitoring technique that has been investigated for many years and has shown promising results [1]. EIT measures the spatial distribution of conductivity by injecting alternating current through electrodes located at the boundary of the body under study; the voltage generated by the injected current is measured by the electrodes at the boundary; these voltages allow the estimation of the conductivity distribution and are mapped to an image with the help of a reconstruction algorithm [11]. In addition, several low-cost EIT systems have been proposed for biomedical applications with high performance [12]. Therefore, this technique is a promising alternative for the diagnosis and monitoring of biological tissues and fluids since they present differences in their dielectric properties.

In bladder volume monitoring, EIT presents many advances that have made it possible to establish a correlation between urine conductivity and bladder volume using the Global Impedance Index (GI) [4], which is calculated from the pixels of the EIT image reconstruction. On the other hand, there are indices based on bioimpedance measurements that do not require image reconstruction algorithms to estimate bladder volumes, such as the IRM (Impedance Ratio Method) [6], VCR (Voltage Change Ratio) [13], and MVCR (Modified Voltage Change Ratio) [7], which, like GI, present a correlation between bioimpedance measurements and bladder volume. The aforementioned methods are highly sensitive to the change in urine conductivity, which occurs due to infections or the patient's diet, so volume estimation with these methods cannot be applied in the long term. For this reason, a method based on global focused impedance (FIM) is proposed in Ref. [7] that allows the estimation of bladder volume independently of urine conductivity, which allows long-term monitoring.

Methods based on bioimpedance measurements are a very good alternative for bladder volume monitoring because they require low-cost equipment and are noninvasive. Considering that GI indices, MRI, VCR, and MVCR are sensitive to urine conductivity, they may also be promising in the study of urinary tract alterations due to infections.

3. Electrical impedance tomography

Figure 1 presents the concept of the EIT, which consists of applying currents (I) on a set of electrodes connected to the boundary ($\partial\Omega$) of a body (Ω); subsequently, the resulting voltages (V) are measured on the remaining electrodes. The mathematical background of the EIT is explained in Ref. [7]; where Maxwell equations and the Faraday and Ampere laws are formulated in the differential form to define the relationship between the admittivity (γ) and the potential on the electrodes (φ) (Eq. 1).

$$\nabla \cdot (\gamma \nabla \varphi) = 0 \tag{1}$$

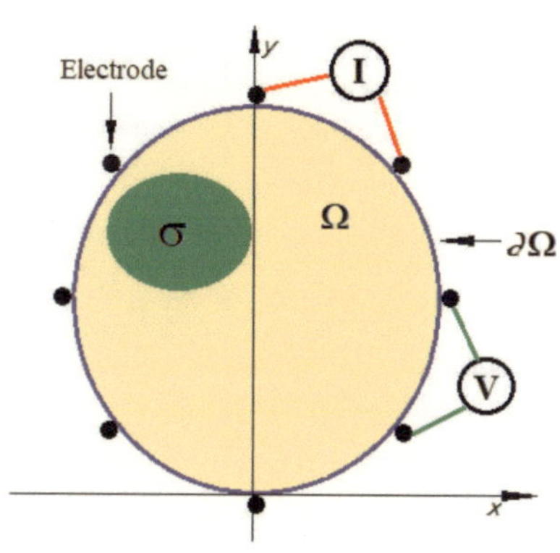

Figure 1.
Conductivity changes detection with EIT.

γ is a complex value $\gamma = \sigma + j\omega\varepsilon$, where σ represents the conductivity $i \triangleq \sqrt{-1}$ is the imaginary unit, ω denotes the angular frequency, and ε is the permittivity. This equation describes the electrical potential inside. Whenever Ω is stimulated with low-frequency currents ($\omega \approx 0$), the following EIT equation is obtained:

$$\nabla \cdot (\sigma \nabla \varphi) = 0 \tag{2}$$

The nonlinear partial differential Eq. 2 has infinite solutions. Particular solutions are obtained by applying either the Dirichlet or Neumann conditions. The former is used when voltages are applied to the boundary electrodes:

$$\varphi(x_i) = v_i \; i = 1, 2, \ldots, m \tag{3}$$

where x_i is a point on $\partial\Omega$ that indicates the position of the electrode i, v_i is the voltage applied to such electrode and m is the total number of electrodes. Neumann conditions are used when currents are injected and drained through the surface electrodes. In such a case:

$$\sigma \nabla \varphi(x_i) \cdot \vec{n} = I_i \; i = 1, 2, \ldots, m \tag{4}$$

where $\vec{n}$ is a unitary vector perpendicular to $\partial\Omega$ in x_i. I_i is the current density through the electrode i and it is positive for the injecting electrode and negative for the draining electrode. Additionally, Kirchoff's current law must be satisfied:

$$\sum_{i=1}^{m} I_i = 0 \tag{5}$$

The solution to the EIT problem is divided into two parts: i) estimate the potentials on the boundary knowing the injected current and assuming a conductivity distribution, this part is called forward problem, and ii) assess the conductivity distribution knowing the injected currents and the measured potentials or inverse problem (**Figure 2**). The forward and inverse problems are detailed below.

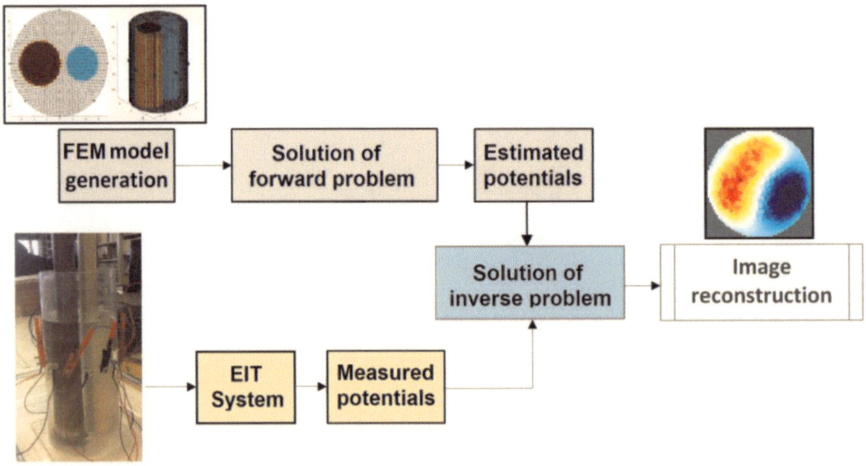

Figure 2.
EIT image reconstruction.

3.1. Forward problem

The forward problem can be solved analytically or numerically. The analytical methods are preferable as computation time is reduced; however, their usage is limited to a few idealized geometries [8]. For numerical solutions, the governing equation is discretized using the finite elements method (FEM) or the generalized FEM (GFEM) [9]. For general geometries and inhomogeneous materials, FEM is well suited to solve the forward problem and is the most used in EIT [10]. In EIT, the approach based on FEM consists of dividing Ω into a finite number of regions of constant conductivity. A relation can be obtained between the voltage measurements on the boundary and the conductivity of such regions (Eq. 6) [11, 12].

$$\Phi = J\sigma \tag{6}$$

where J is known as the sensitivity matrix or Jacobian matrix, which relates the vector of voltage measurements (Φ) with the vector of conductivities (σ). If σ and J are known. Then, the estimation of Φis simple. Considering the variety of methods available in EIDORS (*Electrical Impedance Tomography and Diffuse Optical Tomography Reconstruction Software*).

3.2. Inverse problem

The inverse problem seeks to obtain the conductivity distribution using the potential on the electrodes and the injected currents. To solve the inverse problem is necessary to use a forward model to minimize the difference between the potentials estimated and measured on the boundary (**Figure 2**). There are several approaches to solve the inverse problem, which is ill-posed and is based on linearization and regularization [8]. The conductivity estimation obtained from 3.2 is:

$$J^T\Phi = J^T J\sigma \tag{7}$$

$$\sigma = \left(JJ^T\right)^{-1} J^T\Phi \tag{8}$$

The matrix (JJ^T) is ill-conditioned. The best way to solve this problem is to use regularization techniques [13], which are necessary to obtain a unique solution from an ill-posed EIT problem [14]. Additionally, a regularized solution to the inverse problem improves the reconstructed image quality [15, 16]. For these reasons, many regularization methods, such as Tikhonov [17, 18], Laplace [19], Total Variation [20], Noser [21], Helmholtz-Type [12], projection error propagation-based [15], have been proposed.

4. Volume estimation with bioimpedance

This section presents the GI (Global Impedance), FIM (Focused Impedance Measurement), IRM (Impedance Ratio Method), and VCR (Voltage Change Ratio) techniques, which have been recently proposed for volume estimation in medical applications. GI is defined as the sum of the pixels of an image and as a consequence, it requires to solve the EIT inverse problem. On other hand, the FIM approach does not need the reconstruction matrix; the potential variation is enough to estimate volume.

FIM estimates the impedance of the region of interest by means of two potential measurements mutually perpendicular giving a higher sensitivity in the central region compared to its surroundings [22]. Similar to FIM method, IRM and VCR do not require an image reconstruction algorithm. IRM, proposed in Ref. [6], estimates the volume estimation of an object employing three impedance measurements. On the other hand, VCR requires two voltage measures to estimate the volume [23], although the robustness against the uncertainty of conductivity has not been analyzed. The GI, FIM, IRM, and VCR are explained below.

4.1. Global impedance index

The GI approach is based on reconstructed images of differential EIT (dEIT) in which homogeneous ($\boldsymbol{v_h}$) and nonhomogeneous ($\boldsymbol{v^f_{nh}}$) vector measurements are taken. The superscript f, which ranges from 1 to N_f, indicates the frame. N is the number of voltage measures per frame and is hence the number of elements of vectors $\boldsymbol{v_h}$ and $\boldsymbol{v^f_{nh}}$. Differences between $\boldsymbol{v_h}$ and $\boldsymbol{v^f_{nh}}$ are used in an EIT reconstruction algorithm to calculate changes in the conductivity inside the object under study [5, 24]. Hence, variations in the potential for any frame f are calculated using the following operation:

$$\Delta \mathbf{v^f}(\mathbf{k}) = \frac{\mathbf{v^f_{nh}}(\mathbf{k}) - \mathbf{v_h}(\mathbf{k})}{\mathbf{v_h}(\mathbf{k})}, \mathbf{k} = \mathbf{1}, \mathbf{2}, \ldots \mathbf{N} \tag{9}$$

where $\boldsymbol{\Delta v^f}(\boldsymbol{k})$, $\boldsymbol{v^f_{nh}}(\boldsymbol{k})$ and $\boldsymbol{v_h}(\boldsymbol{k})$ are the k-th elements of the vectors $\boldsymbol{\Delta v^f}$, $\boldsymbol{v^f_{nh}}$ and $\boldsymbol{v_h}$, respectively. To solve the pixel conductivity vector $\boldsymbol{I_f}$, the matrix $\boldsymbol{R^f}$ must be calculated using a differential EIT reconstruction algorithm. $\boldsymbol{R^f}$ has M rows and N columns (M, number of pixels of the conductivity image). Hence, the vectors $\boldsymbol{I^f}$ and $\boldsymbol{\Delta v^f}$ are related by the equation $\boldsymbol{I^f} = \boldsymbol{R^f}\boldsymbol{\Delta v^f}$. GI of dimensionless units is calculated by adding the values of all pixels of $\boldsymbol{I^f}$ for each frame as follows (Eq. 10):

$$\mathbf{GI} = \sum_{\mathbf{f=1}}^{\mathbf{N_f}} \sum_{\mathbf{k=1}}^{\mathbf{N}} \mathbf{I^f} \tag{10}$$

4.2. Focused impedance measurement (FIM)

FIM Method is a technique of impedance measurement that can localize a zone of interest in a volume, eliminating the effects of neighboring regions and using 8, 6, or 4 electrodes [25–27]. FIM shows promising results in gastric monitoring [28], breast tumors [29], and lung ventilation [21]. We propose a modification of the FIM approach using eight electrodes; the classical FIM and modified FIM are explained then.

4.2.1 Classic FIM method

Tetrapolar FIM's are based on the sum of independent measurements of mutually perpendicular and concentric potentials. This is done to detect changes that are generated by the injected current on the equipotential lines inside the object under study. Saha and collaborators [30] show that changes in the conductivity/impedance of the

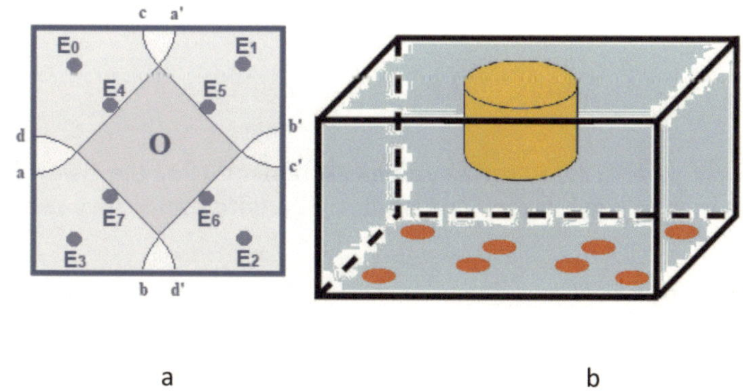

Figure 3.
a) Focused area in an 8-Electrodes FIM arrangement and b) Placement of electrodes on the bladder phantom.

object under study lead to proportional differences in electrical potential between equipotential lines. This assumption remains valid for a constant injected current. The arrangement of electrodes for FIM is shown in **Figure 3**.

When the current is injected through the E0 and E2 electrodes, equipotential lines are represented as $a-a'$ and $b-b'$. Similarly, when current is injected through the E_1 and E_3 electrodes, then the equipotential lines are represented as $c-c'$ and $d-d'$. These potentials are measured on electrodes E_4, E_5, E_6, and E_7, and the focused area O is defined for equipotential lines [31]. Changes in potential are estimated relative to the reference measure P_{ref}, which is the potential when there is no object in the region **O** of **Figure 3**. In this case, the conductivity is homogeneous throughout the cross-section under study. P_{ref} is calculated using Eq. 11 as follows:

$$\mathbf{P_{ref}} = \mathbf{P^0_{4,6}} + \mathbf{P^0_{5,7}} \tag{11}$$

$P^0_{4,6}$ is the difference in potential between the electrodes E_4 and E_5 for the homogeneous configuration (indicated with the superscript o). Similarly, $P^0_{5,7}$ is the difference in potential between the electrodes E_5 and E_7. Hence, given a conductivity change in region O (**Figure 3**), the potential is defined in Eq. 12 as follows:

$$\mathbf{P} = \mathbf{P_{4,6}} + \mathbf{P_{5,7}} \tag{12}$$

	Injection	**Measurement**	
Potentials on internal electrodes	E_0-E_1	$P_{4,5}$	$P_{5,6}$
	E_1-E_2	$P'_{5,6}$	$P_{6,7}$
	E_4-E_5	$P_{6,7}$	
	E_5-E_6	$P_{4,7}$	
Potentials on external electrodes	E_4-E_5	$P_{0,1}$	$P_{1,2}$
	E_5-E_6	$P'_{1,2}$	$P_{2,3}$

Table 1.
Injection and measurement patterns for the proposed FIM approaches.

The variability of potential is then defined as:

$$\Delta \mathbf{P} = \frac{\mathbf{P} - \mathbf{P_{ref}}}{\mathbf{P_{ref}}} \tag{13}$$

The opposite pattern for injection and measurement using the classic FIM approach has been applied in previous studies [32], with promissory results.

4.2.2 Modified FIM method

The modified FIM approach [32] employs adjacent patterns for injection and measurement, using the same electrode arrangement of FIM classic. The electrodes were divided into externals (E_0, E_1, E_2, and E_3) and internals (E_4, E_5, E_6, and E_7) according to the configuration presented in **Figure 3**. **Table 1** shows the injection and measurement electrodes used for the two proposed FIM approaches. In the first proposed FIM approach, FIM-I (I, internal), the variable P of Eq. 13 was equal to $\boldsymbol{P_{int}}$, which is calculated as $\boldsymbol{P_{int}} = \boldsymbol{P_{4,5}} + \boldsymbol{P_{5,6}} + \boldsymbol{P'_{5,6}} + \boldsymbol{P_{6,7}}$. In the second proposed approach, FIM-IE (IE, Internal-External), $\boldsymbol{P} = \boldsymbol{P_{int}} + \boldsymbol{P_{ext}}$ with $\boldsymbol{P_{ext}} = \boldsymbol{P_{0,1}} + \boldsymbol{P'_{1,2}} + \boldsymbol{P_{1,2}} + \boldsymbol{P_{2,3}}$ and $\boldsymbol{P_{int}}$ as for FIM-I. In the previously described FIM-4 approach [32], variable $\boldsymbol{P_{int}} = \boldsymbol{P_{4,7}} + \boldsymbol{P_{6,7}}$. As indicated in **Table 1**, FIM-I requires two injections of current and four measures of voltage, whereas FIM-IE requires four injections of current and eight measures of voltage. In contrast, classic FIM-4 requires two injections of current and two measures of voltage. Pref for each approach is defined as $\boldsymbol{P}$.

4.3. Impedance ratio method (IRM)

IRM relates volume with impedance change. This technique searches the volume estimation robustness against the conductivity variability of the object under study. The three tetrapolar measurements required to calculate the impedance ratio are presented in **Figure 4** [22]. The frontal measurement is used to calculate $Z_f = V_f/I_f$, the backward measurement defines $Z_b = V_b/I_b$, and the side measurement determines $Z_s = V_s/I_s$. The potentials and the currents are measured and injected on boundary electrodes, which are placed in a ring arrangement. The measurements proposed in Ref. [22] present higher sensibility of impedance variations; assuming that the object under study must be close to the electrodes, being that the current densities are the biggest in the vicinity of these. Therefore, the volume increase of the object implies a higher change in the sensitivity of impedance measurements. Eq. 14 defines the IRM.

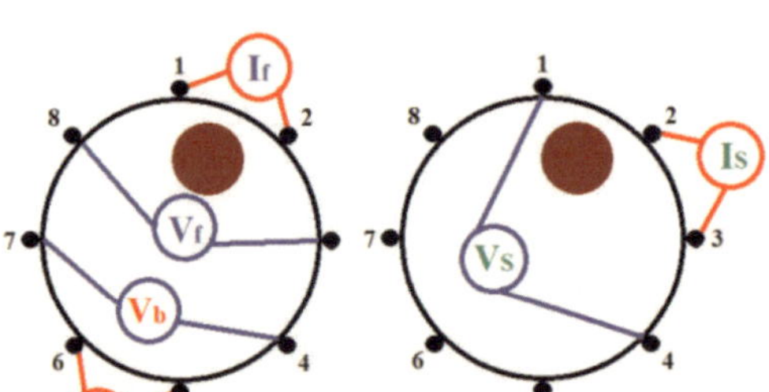

Figure 4.
Injection and measurement of signals for IRM.

$$\mathbf{IRM} = \frac{\mathbf{Z_s - Z_f}}{\mathbf{Z_b - Z_f}} \tag{14}$$

4.4. Voltage change ratio (VCR)

VCR [23] associates the voltage change with the volume of the object under study. This is calculated by considering a reference measurement (V_0), which is obtained when the object studied has the lowest volume. Other potential measurements (V) are taken during the increasing volume to determine the VCR (Eq. 15).

$$\mathbf{VCR} = \frac{|\mathbf{V - V_0}|}{\mathbf{V_0}} \tag{15}$$

The electric potentials are measured by considering the electrode configuration shown in **Figure 5**.

VCR index uses two voltage measurements only, one reference and the other to determine the change in volume; to have redundant voltage measurements, the modified VCR (MVCR) is proposed for Ref. [32]. The MVCR requires 8 voltage measurements, as indicated in **Figure 6**. The MVCR is calculated using Eq. 16.

$$\mathbf{MVCR} = \frac{\sum_{\mathbf{i=8}}^{\mathbf{8}} \frac{|\mathbf{V_i - V_0}|}{\mathbf{V_0}}}{\mathbf{n}} \tag{16}$$

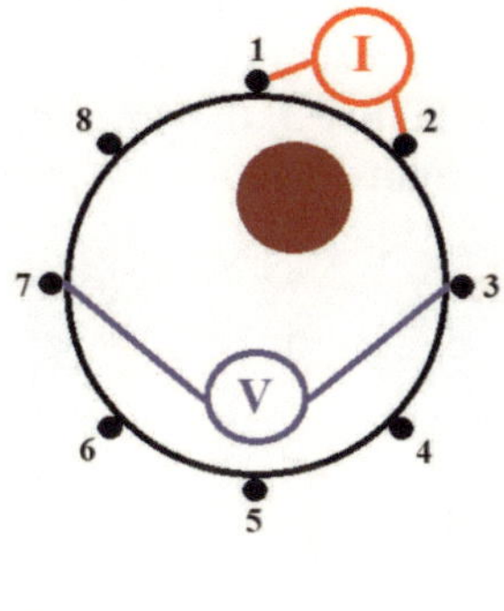

Figure 5.
Injection and measurement of signals for VCR.

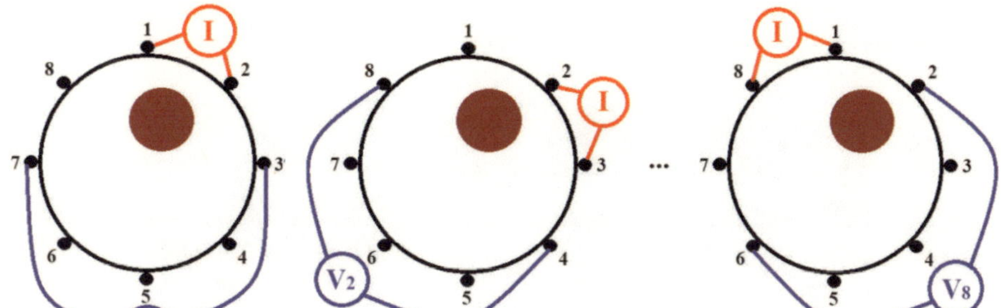

Figure 6.
Injection and measurement of signals for MVCR.

where n is the number of voltage measurements and V_0 is the reference voltage obtained when the current is injected by electrodes 1 and 2 and the studied object has the lowest volume.

5. Results of noninvasive bladder volume monitoring

GI, VCR, MVCR, MVCR, MVCR, IRM, FIM, FIM-I, and FIM-IE indices were employed for *in vitro* experiments to estimate bladder volume employing a bioimpedance measurement system previously designed in Ref. [33, 34], the results of the volume behavior are detailed below.

5.1. Sensitivity of approaches for volume estimation

The sensitivity distribution of an impedance measurement determines the impedance change caused by a given change in conductivity distribution. The sensitivity distribution also establishes the impedance contribution of each region within the area under study. The sensitivity map is the superposition of all the sensitivity distributions corresponding to each measurement. Based on Geselowitz's theorem [35], a study of sensitivity maps for the FIM, GI, VCR, and IRM approaches was performed.

Figure 7 shows that the region center of GI approach has a very low sensitivity, near to zero (represented by white color); on the other hand, the IRM, VCR, and MVCR approaches show a negative sensitivity (blue color). Considering the sensitivity maps, these indices could have the best performance if the object under study is placed near the electrodes, where the sensitivity is high (dark red color).

The sensitivity maps for the approaches based on FIM are generated through the FEM model of the phantom-like **Figure 3**; the green circles represent the location of the electrodes on the phantom. **Figure 8** shows the sensitivity of the approaches base

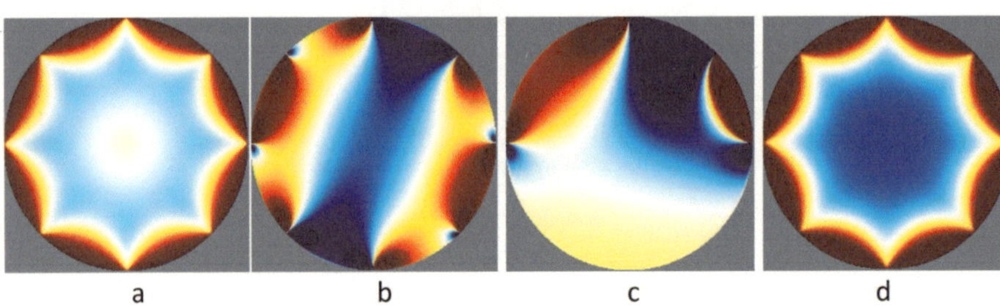

Figure 7.
Sensitivity maps of a) GI, b) IRM, c) VCR, and d) MVCR.

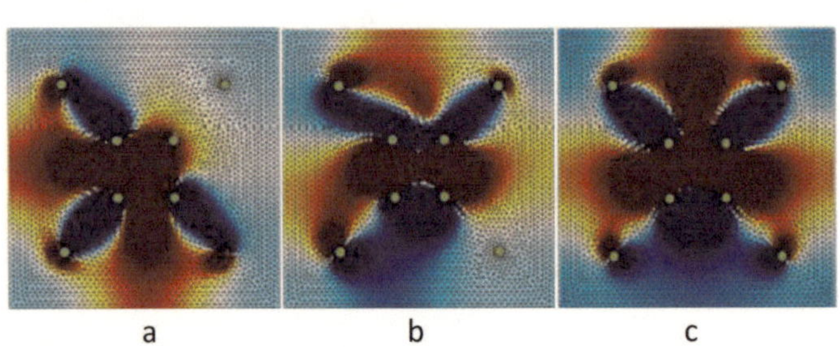

Figure 8.
Sensitivity maps of a) FIM4, b) FIM-I y and c) FIM-IE.

on FIM has greater sensitivity in the central zone than the approaches with the electrodes around the boundary. These results demonstrate that FIM-based approaches are very promising for volume estimation.

5.2. Performance of bladder volume estimation

The experiments *in vitro* to bladder volume estimation showed a linear correlation between abdominal electrical impedance and bladder volume. In Ref. [36], it is evident the linear correlation of GI index with bladder volume. On the other hand, in [mosquera20] the linear relationship positive between GI and volume was confirmed. It was also found that the GI index shows low sensitivity to measurement noise.

On the other hand, the approaches for volume estimation that do not require image reconstruction algorithms show the next results:

- The IRM in *in vitro* experiments does not correlate positively or negatively with the volume [32]. This is because when the object under study is symmetrically located with respect to the electrodes, the front, rear, and side voltages are the same, and as a consequence, the IRM becomes a quotient of noises. This fact makes IRM unsuitable for bladder volume estimation.

- The VCR in Refs. [23, 32] evidence that the median values of the VCR measurements significantly differ for the volume. Also, VCR has a positive correlation with human bladder monitoring. Furthermore.

- The MVCR is an extension of VCR that uses eight voltage measurements to improve robustness against noise, as is evidenced in Ref. [32]. Like VCR, MVCR leads to significant differences in the volume measurement.

The results *in vitro* show that GI, VCR, and MVCR are suitable approaches for volume monitoring when the conductivity of the object under study is unknown but constant. VCR has the highest sensitivity to volume variation, while MVCR had the highest noise robustness. Both VCR and MVCR are easier to implement than GI because they do not require an image reconstruction algorithm.

The studies show that when the volume remains constant, but the conductivity varies, the VCR and MVCR estimates also vary, making it impossible to distinguish between changes in volume and changes in conductivity. GI suffers from the same problem as VCR and MVCR because it is calculated as the sum of the conductivity pixels of an image; as a consequence, a large object with moderate conductivity can have a similar GI as a medium object with high conductivity. The bioimpedance approaches presented in this chapter detect changes in volume when the conductivity of the object under study remains constant. Furthermore, these methods require less computational effort than the GI approach, which is based on differential EIT and as consequence requires to solve the inverse problem.

The FIM-4 approach was proposed in a previous study [22] and comprises two mutually orthogonal tetrapolar measurements to estimate the impedance of an object that is located below the plane formed by the electrodes. Based on FIM-4, a method for organ volume estimation was proposed [37], and it was shown that simulations that are based on finite elements give linear relationships between volumes of study objects and sensitivity, which is defined as the quotient of impedance variation and the distance between electrodes. In addition, *in vitro* experiments demonstrated that the constant that relates volume and sensitivity depends on the conductivity of the object and on its depth with respect to the plane of electrodes. Similarly, FIM-I and FIM-4 approaches depend on the conductivity of the object under study. The experiments with FIM-IE, however, showed a strict dependence on the volume. The main difference between these three FIM approaches is the additional information required to calculate variations of electrical potential. Unlike FIM-I and FIM-4 procedures, FIM-IE is performed by injecting current and measuring the voltage on internal and external electrodes. When current is injected through internal electrodes, voltage is measured at the external electrodes, and *vice versa*.

In *in vivo* experiments it was found that the GI index shows a high variation to changes in urine conductivity [5, 23] making it a method that can be oriented to short-term monitoring. In [23] shows a significantly enhances the sensitivity of the measurement with VCR index, suggesting a better protocol to maximize the value of electrical impedance in monitoring the accumulation of bladder urine.

Each of the present bioimpedance approaches for estimating bladder volumes *in vivo* requires a calibration procedure that begins by emptying the patient's bladder and then using urodynamics to relate bladder volumes to the bioimpedance variable. The resulting equations relate measurements with volumes but are only valid when urine conductivity is equal to that during the calibration phase. Because urine conductivity varies physiologically, it is important to use bioimpedance approaches for which measured variables are independent of urine conductivity. The FIM-IE approach meets these criteria.

The results obtained in studies lead us to conclude that the proposed FIM-IE approach has low sensitivity against conductivity uncertainty, allowing volume monitoring to long-term; contrary to the performance shown by VCR, IRM, and GI indices, which have a high sensibility to conductivity uncertainty as is reported in Refs. [6, 23, 31, 32].

6. Conclusions

Since the methods currently used (cytometry, pressure-flow studies, and electromyography) for urodynamic studies are invasive and can cause irritation, bleeding, infection, urethral fistula, and rupture of the urinary system [10], bioimpedance-based methods are an excellent alternative for bladder monitoring because they do not involve risks due to the use of catheters or probes in the urinary tract. On the other hand, uroflowmetry, being a noninvasive method, is not suitable for the diagnosis of urinary system pathologies [8]; therefore, the use of bioimpedance, being sensitive to urine conductivity and allowing estimation of bladder volume, is a method that could generate a diagnosis of the behavior and state of the urinary system; being a better alternative than uroflowmetry.

Unlike the VCR, MRI, and GI approaches, which are highly sensitive to conductivity changes, FIM-IE is very robust to uncertainty in this variable, making it suitable for long-term bladder volume monitoring. Therefore, FIM-IE is a promising alternative to avoid inappropriate catheterization in patients with loss of voiding sensation and the future, detect vesicoureteral reflux. On the other hand, GI, VCR, and MVCR, being highly sensitive to urine conductivity, may be promising alternatives to test urine conductivity for abnormalities due to bacteria or infections.

Acknowledgements

The authors thank the support of the research group of Automation of Universidad del Cauca (501100005682).

Author details

Víctor Hugo Mosquera
Universidad del Cauca, Popayán, Colombia

*Address all correspondence to: mosquera@unicauica.edu.co

References

[1] Harikumar R, Prabu R, Raghavan S. Electrical impedance tomography (EIT) and its medical applications: A review. International Journal of Software Computer and Engineering. 2013;**3**: 193-198

[2] Dunne E, O'Halloran M, Craven D, Puri P, Frehill P, Loughney S, et al. Detection of vesicoureteral reflux using electrical impedance tomography. IEEE Transactions on Biomedical Engineering. 2018;**66**:2279-2286

[3] Li R, Gao J, Li Y, Wu J, Zhao Z, Liu Y. Preliminary study of assessing bladder urinary volume using electrical impedance tomography. Journal of Medical and Biological Engineering. 2016;**36**:71-79

[4] Schlebusch T, Nienke S, Santos SA, Leonhardt S. Bladder volume estimation from electrical impedance tomography. In: 35th Annual International Conference of the IEEE Engineering in Medicine and Biology Society (EMBC). 2013

[5] Schlebusch T, Leonhardt S. Effect of electrode arrangements on bladder volume estimation by electrical impedance tomography. Journal of Physics: Conference Series. 2013

[6] Schlebusch T, Orschulik J, Malmivuo J, Leonhardt S, Leonhäuser D, Grosse J, et al. Impedance ratio method for urine conductivity - invariant estimation of bladder volume. Journal of Electrical Bioimpedance. 2019;**5**:48-54

[7] Bragos R, Rengifo C, Mosquera V. Robustness of focused and global impedance estimates of bladder volumes against uncertainty of urine conductivity. Biomedical Physics & Engineering Express. 2020;**6**(2): 045008

[8] Abelson BS, Majerus D, Sun B, Gill E, Versi M, Damaser, Ambulatory urodynamic monitoring: State of the art and future directions, Nature Reviews. Urology. 2019;**16**(5):291-301

[9] Li Y, Peng Y, Yang X, Lu S, Gao J, Lin C, et al. Analysis of measurement electrode location in bladder urine monitoring using electrical impedance. Biomedical Engineering Online. 2019;**18**: 34

[10] Salazar MP. El estudio urodinámico, Uroligía Colombiana. 2014;**23**(2):128-1308

[11] Holder DS. Electrical Impedance Tomography: Methods, History and Applications. Institute of Physics Publishing. Boca Raton: CRC Press; 2004

[12] Simini F, Bertemes-Filho P. Bioimpedance in Biomedical Applications and Research. New York: Springer; 2018

[13] Lu L, Liu L, Hu C. Analysis of the electrical impedance tomography algorithm based on finite element method and Tikhonov regularization. In: 2014 International Conference on Wavelet Analysis and Pattern Recognition. 2014

[14] Kantartzis P, Liatsis P. On sparse forward solutions in non-stationary domains for the EIT imaging problem. Annual International Conference of the IEEE Engineering in Medicine and Biology Society. 2011

[15] Zaravi S, Amirfattahi R, Vahdat BV. Expanding 2D block method in two direction by a new formula in EIT. In: 23rd Iranian Conference on Electrical Engineering. 2015

[16] Zaravi S, Amirfattahi R, Vahdat BV, Hassanipour A. Improving 2D block method in electrical impedance tomography. In: 22nd Iranian Conference on Biomedical Engineering (ICBME). 2015

[17] Romano D, Pisa S, Piuzzi E. Implementation of the Newton-Raphson and admittance methods for EIT. International Journal of Bioelectromagnetism. 2010;**12**:12-20

[18] Lionheart WRB. EIT reconstruction algorithms: Pitfalls, challenges and recent developments. Physiological Measurement. 2004;**25**:125

[19] Bera TK, Biswas SK, Rajan K, Nagaraju J. Image reconstruction in Electrical Impedance Tomography (EIT) with projection error propagationbased regularization (PEPR): a practical phantom study. International Conference on Advanced Computing, Networking and Security. 2011

[20] Bera TK, Nagaraju J. A study of practical biological phantoms with simple instrumentation for electrical impedance tomography (\textsc{EIT}). In: de Instrumentation and Measurement Technology Conference, 2009. I2MTC '09. IEEE; 2009

[21] Jin B, Maass P. An analysis of electrical impedance tomography with applications to Tikhonov regularization. ESAIM: Control, Optimisation and Calculus of Variations. 2012;**18**: 1027-1048

[22] Graham BM, Adler A. Electrode placement configurations for 3D EIT. Physiological Measurement. 2007; **28**:S29

[23] Tawil DS, Rye D, Velonaki M. Improved image reconstruction for an EIT-based sensitive skin with multiple internal electrodes. IEEE Transactions on Robotics. 2011;**27**:425-435

[24] Borsic A, Graham BM, Adler A, Lionheart WRB. In vivo impedance imaging with total variation regularization. IEEE Transactions on Medical Imaging. 2009;**29**:44-54

[25] Rabbani KS, Sarker M, Akond MHR, Akter T. Focused impedance measurement (FIM): A new technique with improved zone localization. Annals of the New York Academy of Sciences. 1999;**873**:408-420

[26] Leonhardt S, Cordes A, Plewa H, Pikkemaat R, Soljanik I, Moehring K, et al. Electric impedance tomography for monitoring volume and size of the urinary bladder. Biomedizinische Technik. 2011;**56**:301-307

[27] Schlebusch T, Nienke S, Leonhäuser D, Grosse J, Leonhardt S. Optimal electrode positions to determine bladder volume by bioimpedance spectroscopy. Lecture Notes on Impedance Spectroscopy. 2013;**4**:67-73

[28] Rabbani KS, Karal MAS. A new four-electrode focused impedance measurement (FIM) system for physiological study. Annals of Biomedical Engineering. 2008;**36**: 1072–1077

[29] Abir AR, Rabbani KS-E. Sensitivity study for a 4-electrode focused impedance method (FIM) using finite element method analysis. Bangladesh Journal of Medical Physics. 2015;7

[30] Pettersen FJ, Ferdous H, Kalvøy H, Martinsen ØG, Høgetveit JO. Comparison of four different FIM configurations—A simulation study. Physiological Measurement. 2014;**35**: 1067

[31] Iquebal M, Rabbani KS-E. Correlation of liquid volume in stomach to electrical transfer impedance measurements using FIM. Bangladesh Journal of Medical Physics. 2014;**6**:66-74

[32] Al Amin A, Parvin S, Kadir MA, Tahmid T, Alam SK, Rabbani KS-E. Classification of breast tumour using electrical impedance and machine learning techniques. Physiological Measurement. 2014;**35**:965

[33] Kadir MA, Ahmed SP, Al Quaderi GD, Rahman R, Rabbani KS-E. Application of focused impedance method (FIM) to determine the volume of an object within a volume conductor. In: Proceedings of the 2013 COMSOL Conference, Bangalore, India. 2013

[34] Saha SK, Al-Quaderi GD, Rabbani KS-E. 3D sensitivity of 8-electrode FIM through experimental study in a phantom. Bangladesh Journal of Medical Physics. 2014;**6**:55-65

[35] Rabbani KS-E, Kadir MA. Possible applications of focused impedance method (FIM) in biomedical and other areas of study. Bangladesh journal of Medical Physics. 2013;**4**:67-74

[36] Mosquera VH, Arregui A, Bragós Bardia R, Rengifo CF. Implementation of a low cost prototype for electrical impedance tomography based on the integrated circuit for body composition measurement AFE4300. In: Proceedings of the 11th International Joint Conference on Biomedical Engineering Systems and Technologies (BIOSTEC 2018): January 19–21, 2018: Funchal, Madeira, Portugal. 2018

[37] He W, Ran P, Xu Z, Li B, Li S-N. A 3D visualization method for bladder filling examination based on EIT. Computational and Mathematical Methods in Medicine. 2012;**2012**:9

Section 4

Treatment of Urinary Tract Infections

Chapter 6

Anti-Bacterial Use and Resistance Pattern in Urinary Tract Infections

Tsegaye Melaku Kebede

Abstract

Despite warnings at the beginning of the industrial antibiotic era 70 years ago, antimicrobial resistance (AMR) has become an increasingly intractable health issue. For common bacterial infections, such as urinary tract infections (UTIs), sepsis, and sexually transmitted infections, high rates of antibiotic resistance have been observed globally for the commonly used antibiotics used to treat these infections. This observation indicates that we are facing a shortage of effective antibiotics. This global problem has a significant impact on pregnant women, necessitating urgent multi-sectoral action to achieve the Sustainable Development Goals, with a particular focus on perinatal health. The current chapter focuses on shedding light on the commonly prescribed antibiotics for treating UTI during pregnancy. This chapter also addresses the overview of UTI management and principles of antibiotic regimen selections (effectiveness). Furthermore, it also pointed to the safety concern for selected antibiotics or class of antibiotics primarily used for treatment of UTI. Finally, it provides the details of current tsunami of AR specifically among pregnant women diagnosed with UTI in different settings and countries. In general, without the effective and cautious use of antibiotics, the progress made by the United Nations in reducing maternal and child mortality and morbidity by treating infections during pregnancy, such as UTI, would be at a heightened risk.

Keywords: antibiotics, antimicrobial resistance, pregnancy, urinary tract infections, asymptomatic bacteria

1. Introduction

Despite the fact that both men and women are susceptible to urinary tract infections (UTIs), women are more prone to them due to various factors. These factors include having a shorter urethra compared to men, proximity to the anus which increases the risk of fecal contamination, hormonal changes, and pregnancy [1, 2]. UTIs frequently happen during pregnancy. It is the most typical bacterial illness that pregnant women get. It refers to the invasion of microorganisms and their subsequent growth in any part of the urinary tract system including the kidneys, ureters, bladder, and urethra (**Figure 1**). It can be asymptomatic (positive urine culture in an asymptomatic woman), as well as symptomatic, complicating the diagnostic and antibiotic use process. The three main manifestations of UTI during pregnancy are asymptomatic bacteriuria (ASB), acute cystitis, and pyelonephritis [2, 3]. Approximately, 30%

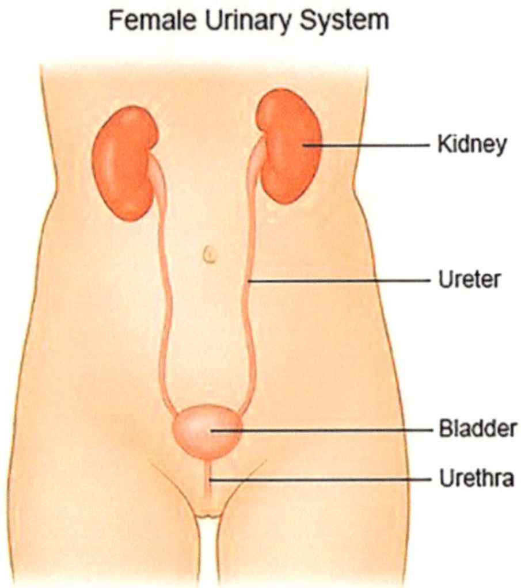

Figure 1.
Female urinary tract system. I declare that there are no copyrights and that the figure is quoted from any other published work for this figure and it is available from the following web link (https://www.drugs.com/cg/urinary-tract-infection-in-women.html).

of women with ASB will experience acute cystitis during their pregnancy, despite the fact that the general incidence of UTI in pregnancy is about 8% [2, 4]. It is of great importance to obstetricians due to its association with significant maternal and perinatal morbidity and mortality.

Pregnancy-related significant bacteriuria is a frequent, serious factor that contributes to maternal and perinatal morbidity and mortality [2, 5]. Bacteriuria during pregnancy raises the mother's risk of anemia, pre-eclampsia, chorioamnionitis, preterm delivery, and postpartum endometritis. Both the fetus and the newborn are at risk of various dangers due to UTI, including preterm birth, stillbirth, perinatal mortality, mental impairment, and developmental delay [1, 3]. The cause is hypothesized to be a combination of direct bacterial endotoxin damage and cerebral hypoperfusion. All are amenable to investigation and treatment, which improves outcomes significantly. However, the rising trend of antimicrobial resistance (AMR) has had a negative impact on the overall outcome of UTI management, as well as neonatal and maternal outcomes [1, 3, 5].

2. Causative pathogens

A meta-analysis of 20 studies from Ethiopia found that 15% of pregnant women receiving prenatal care in various regions had significant bacteriuria [6]. Similar to this, another study from low-income nations found that 13.5% of bacterial uropathogens that cause UTIs were isolated from the urine sample [7]. The majority of the times, the bacteria that cause UTIs in pregnant women are also present in non-pregnant patients. Gram-negative aerobic bacilli that originate in the digestive system are the most frequent cause of UTI. Frequent pathogens responsible for UTI include *Citrobacter*, *Enterobacter*, *Enterococcus*, *Escherichia*, *Klebsiella*, *Proteus*, *Pseudomonas*, *Serratia*, *and Staphylococcus*, which colonize the genitourinary tract

[6, 8, 9]. *Escherichia coli* accounts for 60–80% of all UTIs in pregnancy and is the most prevalent pathogenic bacterium linked to both asymptomatic and symptomatic bacteriuria [6, 7, 10]. Other bacteria identified in UTIs during pregnancy include *Klebsiella pneumoniae* (*K. pneumoniae*), *Staphylococcus aureus*, *coagulase negative Staphylococci*, *Enterobacter* spp., *Pseudomonas aeruginosa*, *Enterococcus* spp., *Proteus mirabilis*, and others [7]. *Klebsiella*, *E. coli*, *Pseudomonas*, and *Proteus* spp. are the most influential gram-negative organisms responsible for UTIs [8]. Among gram-positive bacterial pathogenic strains, *Staphylococcus and Streptococcus* spp. have been found to be the most common bacteria responsible for UTIs [6, 11].

3. Anti-bacterial use in UTI management

Antibiotics are used to treat ASB and acute cystitis. Because ASB is a known risk factor for developing pyelonephritis and having a premature delivery, pregnant women should be screened for it using urine culture and treated with appropriate antimicrobials. Active UTI should be treated as soon as possible after diagnosis; waiting for culture and sensitivity results in the pregnant population is not recommended due to the risk of developing ascending infection [3, 5]. A microbiologic sample must be obtained prior to treatment in order to tailor antibiotic treatment as per the "*Start Smart Then Focus principles*" of antibiotic stewardship. Any treatment decision should be reconsidered once culture and sensitivity reports are available. All women should be checked to ensure that their urine is sterile after treatment for both ASB and active infections [1, 5].

3.1 General principles of anti-bacterial selection

Antibacterial are among the most often prescribed drugs for UTI treatment worldwide, and they are vital to global health. Despite their importance, the development of resistance threatens antibiotics' long-term effectiveness. The overuse and misuse of antibiotics has been the primary cause of antibiotic resistance. The misuse of antibiotics by the general population is a significant risk factor for antibiotic resistance [12], while some studies have also reported that some pregnant women are ignorant of the management of common infections which results in AMR [13].

When the actual cause of the infection and the pattern of resistance are uncertain, empirical antibiotics are chosen [2]. The antibiotics used to treat UTIs are chosen based on a variety of factors, including the relative frequency of uropathogenic organisms, local resistance patterns, levels of observed resistance, the clinical syndrome presented by the patient, and the source of the infection, whether nosocomial or acquired in the community. Therefore, an empirical antibiotic for the treatment of UTIs should be active against gram-positive organisms like *Staphylococcus saprophyticus* and, ideally, *Enterococcus* spp. as well as gram-negative Enterobacteriaceae like *E. coli (E. coli)* and *Klebsiella* spp.

Pregnant women should be treated when bacteriuria is identified (**Table 1**). The choice of antibiotic should address the most common infecting organisms (i.e., gram-negative gastrointestinal organisms). The risk of resistance mutations in the population as well as the specific patient has a significant impact on the selection of empirical antibiotics. Therefore, it is crucial to obtain a comprehensive clinical history since certain patient groups may require early treatment with broad-spectrum antibiotics. Patients who have recently been admitted as inpatients, those who have

Antibiotic	Dosage	Pregnancy category
1. Cephalexin	50 mg two or four times daily	B
2. Erythromycin	250–500 mg four times daily	B
3. Nitrofurantoin	50–100 mg four times daily	B
4. Sulfisoxazole	1 g four times daily	C*
5. Amoxicillin clavulanic acid	250 mg four times daily	B
6. Fosfomycin	One 3g sachet	B
7. Trimethoprimsulfamethoxazole	160/180 mg twice daily	C**

**Contraindicated in pregnant women at term.*
***Avoid during first trimester and at term.*

Table 1.
Antibiotic selection for treatment of UTIs during pregnancy [14, 15].

taken repeated antibiotic courses, and those who live in nursing homes are particularly at risk of contracting infections with multidrug resistant (MDR) organisms. Experts recommend that the choice of antibiotic for empirical treatment should take into account local rates of resistance in uropathogens. Choosing the right antibiotics for pregnant patients with UTIs is critical. It is not only important to choose the right drug, but also consideration should be given to selecting the right dose and treatment duration. When urine culture results are available, antibiotic selection can be tailored based on organism sensitivities. In pregnancy, 1-day antibiotic treatments are not recommended. Instead, 3-day courses are recommended and have been proven to be effective [16, 17]. It is hoped that by effectively treating UTIs, the risk of maternal sepsis, pyelonephritis, preterm labor, and adverse fetal outcomes will be reduced. When selecting antibiotics, potential teratogenicity should be taken into account. The antibiotic should be safe for both the mother and the fetus.

Amoxicillin, ampicillin, ceftriaxone, nitrofurantoin, and trimethoprim-sulfamethoxazole are common antibiotics. Due to conflicting studies on teratogenicity, fluoroquinolones are not recommended as first-line treatment in pregnancy [18]. However, it is reasonable to take this class of medication with resistant or recurrent infections because short courses are unlikely to be detrimental to the fetus. Historically, ampicillin was the drug of choice, but *E. coli* has become increasingly resistant to ampicillin in recent years. Around 20–30% of *E. coli* isolated from urine in an outpatient environment have ampicillin resistance [17]. The high urine concentration of nitrofurantoin makes it a good choice. Cephalosporins, on the other hand, are well tolerated and effectively treat the key microorganisms. Fosfomycin is a novel antibiotic that is administered in a single dose. Sulfonamides are safe to use during the first and second trimesters, but they increase the risk of kernicterus in the third trimester, especially in preterm infants. Other common antibiotics (for example, fluoroquinolones and tetracyclines) should not be used during pregnancy due to potential fetal toxicity [17, 18].

Usually, a 7- to 10-day course of antibiotics is enough to completely get rid of the infection(s). However, shorter treatment durations, including 1-day therapy, have been recommended by some experts. There is still debate over whether pregnant individuals should take shorter antibiotic rounds of treatment. In a clinical trial conducted by Masterton et al. [14], it was found that for isolates that were sensitive to ampicillin, the cure rate reached up to 88% with a single 3 g dosage of ampicillin.

According to several other studies, cure rates for bacteriuria ranged from 50% to 78% when amoxicillin, cephalexin, or nitrofurantoin was given as a single dosage [15, 19]. Fosfomycin is effective when taken as a single, 3g sachet [20, 21]. Further research is necessary to evaluate whether a shorter course of other antibiotics would be as successful as the standard treatment duration for UTIs because other antibiotics have not been well studied for use in UTIs [15]. Following the completion of the treatment regimen, a repeat culture should be obtained to document successful bacteriuria eradication [19].

3.2 Anti-bacterial safety concern in pregnancy

Due to the excretion of several drugs through the kidneys, they may prove beneficial in treating UTI due to their potential to concentrate in the renal system. However, where the safety of the fetus or newborn is a concern, the pregnancy state prohibits the use of certain antibiotics. When the benefits outweigh the risks, the antibiotic can be used if no other option is available. As a result, the choice of antibiotics during pregnancy may be limited in comparison to the general population due to the risk of teratogenicity, or harm to the developing fetus. For example, trimethoprim is avoided in the first trimester due to a risk of neural tube abnormalities, and the danger of hemolysis prevents the use of nitrofurantoin at term [22].

3.2.1 Sulfa derivatives and nitrofurantoin

Recent research suggests that using nitrofurantoin and sulfa derivatives during the first trimester of pregnancy increases the risk of congenital disabilities. While acknowledging the severe limitations of these trials, current guidelines advise against using these drugs during the first trimester of pregnancy when alternatives are available [23]. However, due to the potential serious implications of untreated UTIs during pregnancy, it is considered reasonable to use these drugs when necessary, as the benefits significantly outweigh the associated risks. There are additional warnings regarding these two types of antibiotics. Patients with glucose 6 phosphate dehydrogenase (G6PD) deficiency should not be prescribed sulfa derivatives or nitrofurantoin as these medications can precipitate hemolysis. Trimethoprim sulfamethoxazole (TMP-SMX) should be avoided in the late third trimester due to the potential risk for the development of kernicterus in the newborn after birth. If sufficient serum levels are present at the time of delivery, sulfonamides pose a risk of neonatal jaundice. The addition of trimethoprim increases activity but trimethoprim inhibits folate synthesis, which is crucial for preventing neural tube deformities. Trimethoprim alone or TMP-SMX combinations should be avoided in the first trimester as well as after 32 weeks gestation [23].

3.2.2 Beta lactam antibiotics

Usually, data on pregnancy safety is very limited, which raises serious concerns during prescription. Furthermore, many studies on the safe use of antibiotics during pregnancy are inconclusive or require more evidence. Nevertheless, beta-lactam antibiotics, known for their extensive use without causing significant adverse effects on fetuses, continue to be the safest choice during pregnancy. Due to their mechanism of action, which involves targeting the bacterial cell wall—a structure exclusive to bacteria—beta-lactam antibiotics exhibit higher selective toxicity. As a

4. Anti-bacterial resistance pattern in pregnant women diagnosed with UTI

While antibiotics are highly effective at treating UTIs, they are also associated with AMR, which is a global health threat. AMR refers to the evolution of microorganisms to develop resistance to antimicrobial treatment. AMR kept rising as a result of the worldwide rapid growth of resistant microorganisms [47]. Recent World Health Organization (WHO) surveillance data from 22 high- and low-income countries show a high level of AMR to numerous bacterial infections, with *E. coli* and *K. pneumoniae* being the most common resistant pathogens [48]. Additionally, a meta-analysis of 23 studies from various parts of the world revealed that pregnant women with substantial bacteriuria had a high incidence of Enterobacteriaceae that produce extended-spectrum beta-lactamases (ESBLs) [49]. Uropathogenic resistance to third-generation cephalosporin, amoxicillin, and other antibiotics in pregnant women, particularly in Africa, poses a significant barrier to the treatment of UTI during pregnancy [49, 50]. Increases in bacterial resistance and the emergence of antibiotic-resistant diseases are closely correlated with the prescription and use of antibiotics.

Resistant infections are difficult to treat and have a high morbidity and mortality rate. There is evidence to suggest that antibiotics to treat UTIs are overused in pregnant women [51], potentially leading to an increase in resistant UTIs. Resistant UTIs can be particularly concerning during pregnancy [2]. Treating such infections can already be challenging, but the additional complexity of ensuring the safety of both the woman and the fetus adds further difficulty in the context of pregnancy. In the majority of low-income nations, routine antibiotic susceptibility testing is a significant problem [52]. As a result, most pregnant women are treated with an unnecessary antibiotic, which contributes to the emergence of resistant pathogens [53]. Considering this, it is necessary to monitor the use of antibiotics in pregnancy to optimize prescribing and consumption of these valuable medicines and facilitate antimicrobial stewardship in antenatal care.

Antibiotic resistance has led to significant challenges in treating UTI [54]. Different studies from low-income countries showed high level of drug resistance. For example, the pooled analysis from Ethiopia showed gram-negative bacteria such as *E. coli* was highly resistant to amoxicillin (81%) and ampicillin (80%) [6]. Similarly, report from Ghana showed that 79.3% of *E. coli* were ampicillin resistant [55]. A multicenter investigation in Tanzania found higher resistance of *E. coli* to ampicillin (94.5%) and cotrimoxazole (88.8%) [56]. In contrast, a meta-analysis in Ethiopia revealed that relatively lower percentage (40%) of *E. coli* isolates were cotrimoxazole-resistant [6]. The results showed that *E. coli* was less resistant to the antibiotics nitrofurantoin (19%), ceftriaxone (20%), and ciprofloxacin (21%). Similarly, Emami et al. [50] reported that *E. coli* was 22% resistant to nitrofurantoin. The Ethiopian data report by [6] showed that 83% of the *E. coli* isolates were MDR and 19% were ESBL producers. This resistance burden is expected to be more prevalent in low resource settings like countries in Sub-Saharan Africa. For example, recent data from Ethiopia showed significantly high burden of anti-bacterial resistance among pregnant women diagnosed with UTI (**Figures 2** and **3**) [6]. Similar findings were reported in another meta-analysis by Mansouri et al. [49] and a study by Sekikubo et al. [53], where 17% and 18% of the *E. coli* strains identified from pregnant women with UTIs were ESBL producers, respectively.

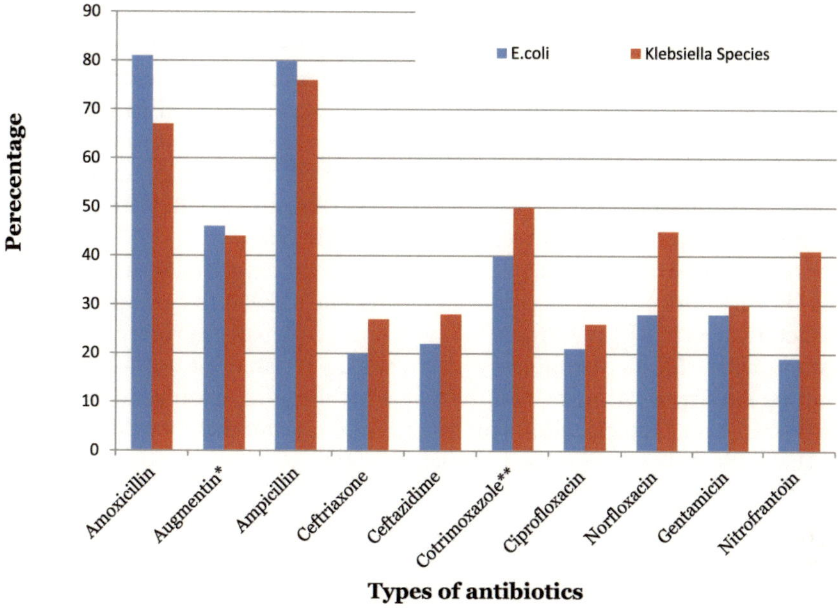

Figure 2.
Pattern of antimicrobial resistance of gram-negative bacteria among pregnant women in Ethiopia [6], pp. 663–686.

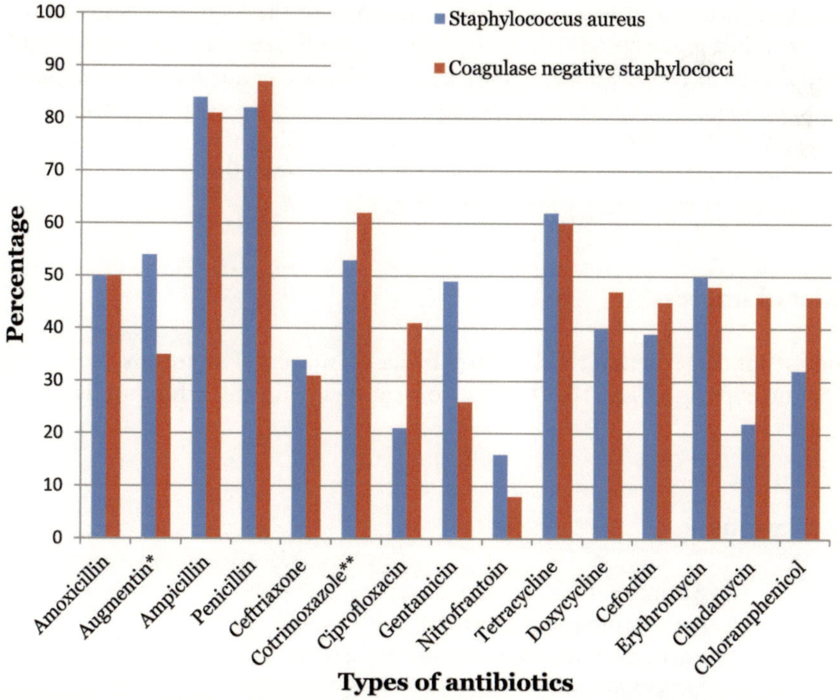

Figure 3.
Pattern of antimicrobial resistance of gram-positive bacteria among pregnant women in Ethiopia [6], pp. 663–686.

Similarly, different studies showed significantly high burden of gram-positive resistance pathogen to common antibiotics. For instance, a meta-analysis from Ethiopia [6] revealed that 89% of the *S. aureus* isolates from urine samples of pregnant women with severe bacteriuria were MDR. Similarly, a study from Nigeria [57] which found that *S. aureus* isolated from urine samples of pregnant women was 90% resistant to cefoxitin, vancomycin, tetracycline, and cotrimoxazole. Another study by Asmat et al. [58] revealed that all *S. aureus* isolates were also MDR, with resistance to tetracycline, doxycycline, tobramycin, and pipemidic acid.

Unsurprisingly, multidrug-resistant bacteria such as extended spectrum beta-lactamases (ESBL), vancomycin-resistant Enterococci (VRE), and carbapenem-resistant Enterobacteriaceae (CRE) have increased and spread globally in recent years [59]. Understanding the local epidemiology of multidrug-resistant bacteria is critical for determining empirical antimicrobial therapy. Furthermore, in order to combat these multidrug-resistant bacteria, clinicians and scientists around the world are working against the clock to develop new antibiotics [59, 60].

5. Conclusion

In conclusion, significant bacteriuria is common among pregnant women. Resistance to commonly used antibiotics is widespread among common bacteria (*E. coli*, *Klebsiella* species, *Staphylococcus* species) causing UTIs in pregnant women. The high occurrence of bacteriuria in pregnant women should serve as a warning to health workers to screen for bacteriuria at least once using urine culture during antenatal care and treat if urine cultures are positive. Because of the high prevalence of drug resistance, it is imperative to create an effective infection control and stewardship program as well as routine epidemiological surveillance of antibiotic resistance. Failure to do so not only prolongs sickness and exposes patients to complications, but also contributes to the development of bacterial resistance as a result of injudicious antibiotic use. It is shown that a high number of antibiotics could be used with relatively great safety during pregnancy to treat UTI.

Conflict of interest

The author declares that there is no conflict of interest. The author declares that there are no copyrights and that the figure is quoted from any other published work in the figures.

Abbreviations

AMR	Antimicrobial resistance
ASB	Asymptomatic bacteriuria
CRE	Carbapenem-resistant Enterobacteriaceae
E. coli	*Escherichia coli*
ESBL	Extended spectrum beta lactamase
FDA	Food and drug authority
G6PD	Glucose 6 phosphate dehydrogenase
K. pneumoniae	*Klebsiella pneumoniae*

DOI: http://dx.doi.org/10.5772/intechopen.111817

MDR	Multidrug resistance
MIC	Minimum inhibitory concentration
TMP-SMX	Trimethoprim sulfamethoxazole
UTI	Urinary tract infection
WHO	World Health Organization

Author details

Tsegaye Melaku Kebede
Institute of Health, Jimma University, Jimma, Ethiopia

*Address all correspondence to: tsegish.melaku@gmail.com; tsegaye.melaku@ju.edu.et

References

[1] Hooton TM, Stamm W. Urinary Tract Infections and Asymptomatic Bacteriuria in Pregnancy. UpToDate. Waltham, MA: UpToDate; 2010

[2] McCormick T, Ashe RG, Kearney PM. Urinary tract infection in pregnancy. The Obstetrician & Gynaecologist. 2008;**10**(3):156-162

[3] Kalinderi K et al. Urinary tract infection during pregnancy: current concepts on a common multifaceted problem. Journal of Obstetrics and Gynaecology. 2018;**38**(4):448-453

[4] Griebling TL. Urinary tract infection in women. Urologic Diseases in America. 2007;7:587-619

[5] Millar LK, Cox SM. Urinary tract infections complicating pregnancy. Infectious Disease Clinics. 1997;**11**(1):13-26

[6] Chelkeba L et al. Bacterial profile and antimicrobial resistance patterns of common bacteria among pregnant women with bacteriuria in Ethiopia: a systematic review and meta-analysis. Archives of Gynecology and Obstetrics. 2022;**306**(3):1-24. DOI: 10.1007/s00404-021-06365-4

[7] Belete MA, Saravanan M. A systematic review on drug resistant urinary tract infection among pregnant women in developing countries in Africa and Asia; 2005-2016. Infection and Drug Resistance. 2020;**13**:1465

[8] Ahmed SS et al. Uropathogens and their antimicrobial resistance patterns: Relationship with urinary tract infections. International Journal of Health Sciences. 2019;**13**(2):48

[9] Wojno KJ et al. Multiplex PCR based urinary tract infection (UTI) analysis compared to traditional urine culture in identifying significant pathogens in symptomatic patients. Urology. 2020;**136**:119-126

[10] Azami M et al. The etiology and prevalence of urinary tract infection and asymptomatic bacteriuria in pregnant women in Iran: a systematic review and meta-analysis. BMC Urology. 2019;**19**(1):1-15

[11] Gessese YA et al. Urinary pathogenic bacterial profile, antibiogram of isolates and associated risk factors among pregnant women in Ambo town, Central Ethiopia: a cross-sectional study. Antimicrobial Resistance & Infection Control. 2017;**6**(1):1-10

[12] Melander E, Jönsson G, Mölstad S. Frequency of penicillin-resistant pneumococci in children is correlated to community utilization of antibiotics. The Pediatric Infectious Disease Journal. 2000;**19**(12):1172-1177

[13] Chavkin W et al. National survey of the states: policies and practices regarding drug-using pregnant women. American Journal of Public Health. 1998;**88**(1):117-119

[14] Masterton R, Evans D, Strike P. Single-dose amoxycillin in the treatment of bacteriuria in pregnancy and the puerperium-a controlled clinical trial. BJOG: An International Journal of Obstetrics & Gynaecology. 1985;**92**(5):498-505

[15] Patterson TF, Andriole VT. Bacteriuria in pregnancy. Infectious Disease Clinics of North America. 1987;**1**(4):807-822

[16] Jolley JA, Wing DA. Pyelonephritis in pregnancy. Drugs. 2010;**70**(13):1643-1655

[17] da Mata N et al. Pharmacodynamics and pharmacokinetics of anti-infective agents in pregnant women. Pregnancy and Anti-Infective Agents. 2020;**4**:21

[18] Lamont HF, Blogg HJ, Lamont RF. Safety of antimicrobial treatment during pregnancy: a current review of resistance, immunomodulation and teratogenicity. Expert Opinion on Drug Safety. 2014;**13**(12):1569-1581

[19] LeFevre M. Urinary tract infections during pregnancy. American Family Physician. 2000;**61**(3):713-720

[20] Bayrak Ö et al. Is single-dose fosfomycin trometamol a good alternative for asymptomatic bacteriuria in the second trimesterof pregnancy? International Urogynecology Journal. 2007;**18**(5):525-529

[21] Estebanez A et al. Fosfomycin in a single dose versus a 7-day course of amoxicillin–clavulanate for the treatment of asymptomatic bacteriuria during pregnancy. European Journal of Clinical Microbiology & Infectious Diseases. 2009;**28**(12):1457-1464

[22] Rizvi M et al. Rising prevalence of antimicrobial resistance in urinary tract infections during pregnancy: necessity for exploring newer treatment options. Journal of Laboratory Physicians. 2011;**3**(02):98-103

[23] Practice C.o.O., Committee Opinion No. 717. Sulfonamides, nitrofurantoin, and risk of birth defects. Obstetrics & Gynecology. 2017;**130**(3):e150-e152

[24] Czeizel AE et al. Augmentin treatment during pregnancy and the prevalence of congenital abnormalities: a population-based case-control teratologic study. European Journal of Obstetrics & Gynecology and Reproductive Biology. 2001;**97**(2):188-192

[25] Czeizel AE et al. A population-based case-control teratologic study of ampicillin treatment during pregnancy. American Journal of Obstetrics and Gynecology. 2001;**185**(1):140-147

[26] Czeizel AE et al. Use of cephalosporins during pregnancy and in the presence of congenital abnormalities: a population-based, case-control study. American Journal of Obstetrics and Gynecology. 2001;**184**(6):1289-1296

[27] Czeizel AE, Rockenbauer M, Olsen J. Use of antibiotics during pregnancy. European Journal of Obstetrics & Gynecology and Reproductive Biology. 1998;**81**(1):1-8

[28] Shetty N, Shulmant R, Scott G. An audit of first generation cephalosporin usage. Journal of Hospital Infection. 1999;**41**(3):229-232

[29] Ilett KF et al. Transfer of probenecid and cephalexin into breast milk. Annals of Pharmacotherapy. 2006;**40**(5):986-989

[30] Jack DB. Pharmacokinetic data on cephalosporins and other anti-infective agents. In: Jack DB, editor. Handbook of Clinical Pharmacokinetic Data. Palgrave Macmillan, London: Springer; 1992. pp. 89-94

[31] Kalman D, Barriere SL. Review of the pharmacology, pharmacokinetics, and clinical use of cephalosporins. Texas Heart Institute Journal. 1990;**17**(3):203

[32] Matsuda S et al. Pharmacokinetic and clinical studies on imipenem/cilastatin sodium in the perinatal period. A study of imipenem/cilastatin sodium

in the perinatal co-research group. The Japanese Journal of Antibiotics. 1988;**41**(11):1731-1741

[33] Heikkilä A, Erkkola R. Review of β-lactam antibiotics in pregnancy. Clinical Pharmacokinetics. 1994;**27**(1):49-62

[34] Dashe JS, Gilstrap LC III. Antibiotic use in pregnancy. Obstetrics and Gynecology Clinics of North America. 1997;**24**(3):617-629

[35] Dinsmoor MJ, Gibbs RS. The role of the newer antimicrobial agents in obstetrics and gynecology. Clinical Obstetrics and Gynecology. 1988;**31**(2):423-434

[36] Chimura T et al. Clinical studies on aztreonam in perinatal use. The Japanese Journal of Antibiotics. 1990;**43**(4):696-699

[37] Stein GE. Single-dose treatment of acute cystitis with fosfomycin tromethamine. Annals of Pharmacotherapy. 1998;**32**(2):215-219

[38] Patel SS, Balfour JA, Bryson HM. Fosfomycin tromethamine. Drugs. 1997;**53**(4):637-656

[39] Saravanos K, Duff P. The quinolone antibiotics. Obstetrics and Gynecology Clinics of North America. 1992;**19**(3):529-537

[40] Loebstein R et al. Pregnancy outcome following gestational exposure to fluoroquinolones: a multicenter prospective controlled study. Antimicrobial Agents and Chemotherapy. 1998;**42**(6):1336-1339

[41] Hooton TM, Stamm WE. Diagnosis and treatment of uncomplicated urinary tract infection. Infectious Disease Clinics. 1997;**11**(3):551-581

[42] Mahadevan U, McConnell RA, Chambers CD. Drug safety and risk of adverse outcomes for pregnant patients with inflammatory bowel disease. Gastroenterology. 2017;**152**(2):451-462.e2

[43] Kaplan YC, Koren G. Use of ciprofloxacin during breastfeeding. Canadian Family Physician. 2015;**61**(4):343-344

[44] José M, Elisa G-V, Jordi V. Macrólidos, cetólidos y estreptograminas. Enfermedades infecciosas y microbiologia clinica. 2003;**21**(4):200-208

[45] Einarson A et al. A prospective controlled multicentre study of clarithromycin in pregnancy. American Journal of Perinatology. 1998;**15**(9):523-525

[46] Kamath P, Kamath A, Ullal SD. Liver injury associated with drug intake during pregnancy. World Journal of Hepatology. 2021;**13**(7):747

[47] Aslam B et al. Antibiotic resistance: a rundown of a global crisis. Infection and Drug Resistance. 2018;**11**:1645

[48] Chand KS, Kapoor P. Two case reports of integrated management of antibiotic-resistant urinary tract infection. Homeopathy. 2020;**109**(2):097-106

[49] Mansouri F et al. Extended-spectrum beta-lactamase (ESBL)-producing Enterobacteriaceae and urinary tract infections in pregnant/postpartum women: a systematic review and meta-analysis. International Journal of Clinical Practice. 2019;**73**(12):e13422. DOI: 10.1111/ijcp.13422

[50] Emami A, Javanmardi F, Pirbonyeh N. Antibiotic resistant profile

of asymptomatic bacteriuria in pregnant women: a systematic review and meta-analysis. Expert Review of Anti-Infective Therapy. 2020;**18**(8):807-815

[51] Kaye KS, Pogue JM. Infections caused by resistant gram-negative bacteria: epidemiology and management. Pharmacotherapy: The Journal of Human Pharmacology and Drug Therapy. 2015;**35**(10):949-962

[52] Seni J et al. Multicentre evaluation of significant bacteriuria among pregnant women in the cascade of referral healthcare system in North-Western Tanzania: bacterial pathogens, antimicrobial resistance profiles and predictors. Journal of Global Antimicrobial Resistance. 2019;**17**:173-179

[53] Sekikubo M et al. Antibiotic overconsumption in pregnant women with urinary tract symptoms in Uganda. Clinical Infectious Diseases. 2017;**65**(4):544-550

[54] Waller TA et al. Urinary tract infection antibiotic resistance in the United States. Primary Care: Clinics in Office Practice. 2018;**45**(3):455-466

[55] Akua FO et al. Escherichia coli Bcteriuria in pregnant women in Ghana: antibiotic resistance pattern, virulence factors and resistant genetic markers. 2018. BioRxiv:317065. DOI: 10.1101/317065

[56] Kaduma J et al. Urinary tract infections and preeclampsia among pregnant women attending two hospitals in Mwanza City, Tanzania: a 1:2 matched case-control study. BioMed Research International. 2019;**2019**. DOI: 10.1155/2019/3937812

[57] Onanuga A, Omeje MC, Eboh DD. Carriage of multi-drug resistant urobacteria by asymptomatic pregnant women in Yenagoa, Bayelsa State, Nigeria. African Journal of Infectious Diseases. 2018;**12**(2):14-20

[58] Asmat U, Mumtaz MZ, Malik A. Rising prevalence of multidrug-resistant uropathogenic bacteria from urinary tract infections in pregnant women. Journal of Taibah University Medical Sciences. 2021;**16**(1):102-111

[59] Petty LA et al. Overview of meropenem-vaborbactam and newer antimicrobial agents for the treatment of carbapenem-resistant Enterobacteriaceae. Infection and Drug Resistance. 2018;**11**:1461

[60] Wagenlehner FM, Naber KG. Cefiderocol for treatment of complicated urinary tract infections. The Lancet Infectious Diseases. 2019;**19**(1):22-23

Chapter 7

New Strategies for the Prevention of Urinary Tract Infections by Uropathogenic *Escherichia coli*

Juan Xicohtencatl-Cortes, Sara A. Ochoa, Ariadnna Cruz-Córdova, Marco A. Flores-Oropeza and Rigoberto Hernández-Castro

Abstract

Uropathogenic *Escherichia coli* (UPEC) is the leading causal agent of urinary tract infections (UTIs), which present high morbidity and limitations in antibiotic treatments. UTIs can also manifest as recurrent (RUTIs) in children and adults and represent a severe public health problem, mainly because there are no treatment and control alternatives that are 100% effective. Patients with RUTIs have a decreased quality of life and are prone to significant complications of UTIs, such as pyelonephritis and urosepsis. Recently, we described UPEC clinical strains related to UTI that have a high profile of antibiotic resistance [multidrug-resistant (MDR) and extensively drug-resistant (XDR)] and genes encoding several fimbrial adhesins, such as FimH of type 1 fimbriae, PapG of fimbriae P, and CsgA of Curli fimbriae. Recently, the expression of fimbrial adhesins (FimH, CsgA, and PapG) was shown to be involved in the release of the interleukins (IL) 6 and IL-8 *in vitro*. This work aims to present a broad overview and description of the pathogenic attributes of UPEC, including the infection processes, pathogenicity mechanisms, and host immune responses, as well as an integral perspective to generate new studies that would contribute to the implementation of preventive strategies against UTI.

Keywords: uropathogenic *Escherichia coli*, resistance, adherence, vaccine, prevention

1. Introduction

Urinary tract infections (UTIs) represent a severe public health problem, and 150 million cases occur annually worldwide. In addition, approximately 40% of women and 12% of men experience at least one UTI event with symptoms in their lives. Different epidemiological data have indicated that a quarter of women who have developed a UTI may present a recurrent infection within six to 12 months [1].

Despite the regular flow of urine, the physiological barriers, and the different defense mechanisms of the host, the urinary tract constitutes one of the most common sites affected by bacterial infection. UTIs originate from the presence of microorganisms in the urinary tract in sufficient quantity to cause clinical symptoms. Depending on the characteristics of the infectious process and the affected site, UTIs can be defined as lower UTIs (cystitis) and uncomplicated pyelonephritis; complicated UTIs with or without pyelonephritis, urinary sepsis or urethritis; and UTIs considered to be special disease types (prostatitis, epididymitis, and orchitis). Depending on the evolution time, they are considered acute and chronic due to symptomatic and asymptomatic clinical manifestations (**Figure 1**) [2].

From a microbiological perspective, UTIs exist when pathogenic microorganisms are detected in the urine, urethra, bladder, kidney, or prostate. Regarding the pathogenesis of UTIs, most begin as a bladder infection (cystitis) caused by bacteria that colonize the perineum, later reach the urethra, and finally colonize the bladder. In cases where cystitis is not properly treated, the bacteria that colonize the bladder can ascend through the ureters and cause pyelonephritis or acute kidney infection, which can even lead to permanent kidney damage (**Figure 1**). In severe cases of pyelonephritis, the bacteria infect the epithelium and endothelium in the kidney and thereby pass into the bloodstream (bacteremia) and cause systemic infection and sepsis, which can result in fatal consequences for the affected individual [3, 4]. The UTI diagnosis, in general, is attained using a general urine test, looking for the presence of leukocyte esterase, the reduction of nitrates to nitrites, the inflammatory cell count (more than 10 cells), and the presence of bacteria. This test has a sensitivity of 75–90% and a specificity of 70–82%. However, urine culture has the limitation of the ability to have an adequate sample for the process; if the urine is obtained from a collection bag, the sensitivity and specificity are very low, since the samples may be contaminated. Additionally, if urine is obtained by catheter, the sensitivity and specificity are greater than 70%, while with collection by suprapubic puncture, the presence of any number of bacterial colonies allows us to ensure the diagnosis. The number of colony-forming units (CFU) necessary to establish the diagnosis of a UTI depends on the type of sample obtained, although it has been considered that this number should be equal to or greater than 10^5 CFU/mL. In the diagnosis, procedures such as excretory urography with a voiding histogram and ultrasound can be used, and this approach has gradually displaced the previous procedure [5].

UTIs are caused by gram-negative and gram-positive uropathogens, in order of importance: uropathogenic *E. coli* (UPEC), *Klebsiella pneumoniae*, *Staphylococcus saprophyticus*, *Enterococcus faecalis*, group B β-hemolytic *Streptococcus*, *Proteus mirabilis*, *Pseudomonas aeruginosa*, *Staphylococcus aureus*, and *Candida spp*. [6]. UPEC is the causal agent of more than 80% of community-acquired cystitis, more than 70% of unreported acute pyelonephritis, and 3.6–12% of UTIs complicated by urosepsis [7].

E. coli is a commensal bacterium of the intestinal tract of humans and animals and is widely distributed in hospital units. Several clinical features of intestinal infections are caused by extraintestinal *E. coli* (ExPEC) and diarrheagenic *E. coli* pathotypes [8–10]. Meanwhile, the diarrheagenic pathotypes of *E. coli* tend to produce self-limited infections. ExPEC causes infections in various nonintestinal anatomical sites, rapidly progressing to complicated infections of bacteremia, sepsis, and meningitis, which requires immediate antibiotic treatment. In addition, ExPECs have independent virulence factors that confer their ability to survive diverse ecological niches and cause damage [10, 11]. Various lineages of ExPEC have been responsible for infections in humans and animals worldwide [12]. The ExPEC pathotypes recognized so far are neonatal meningitis *E. coli* (NMEC), sepsis-associated *E. coli* (SEPEC), avian

DOI: http://dx.doi.org/10.5772/intechopen.108911

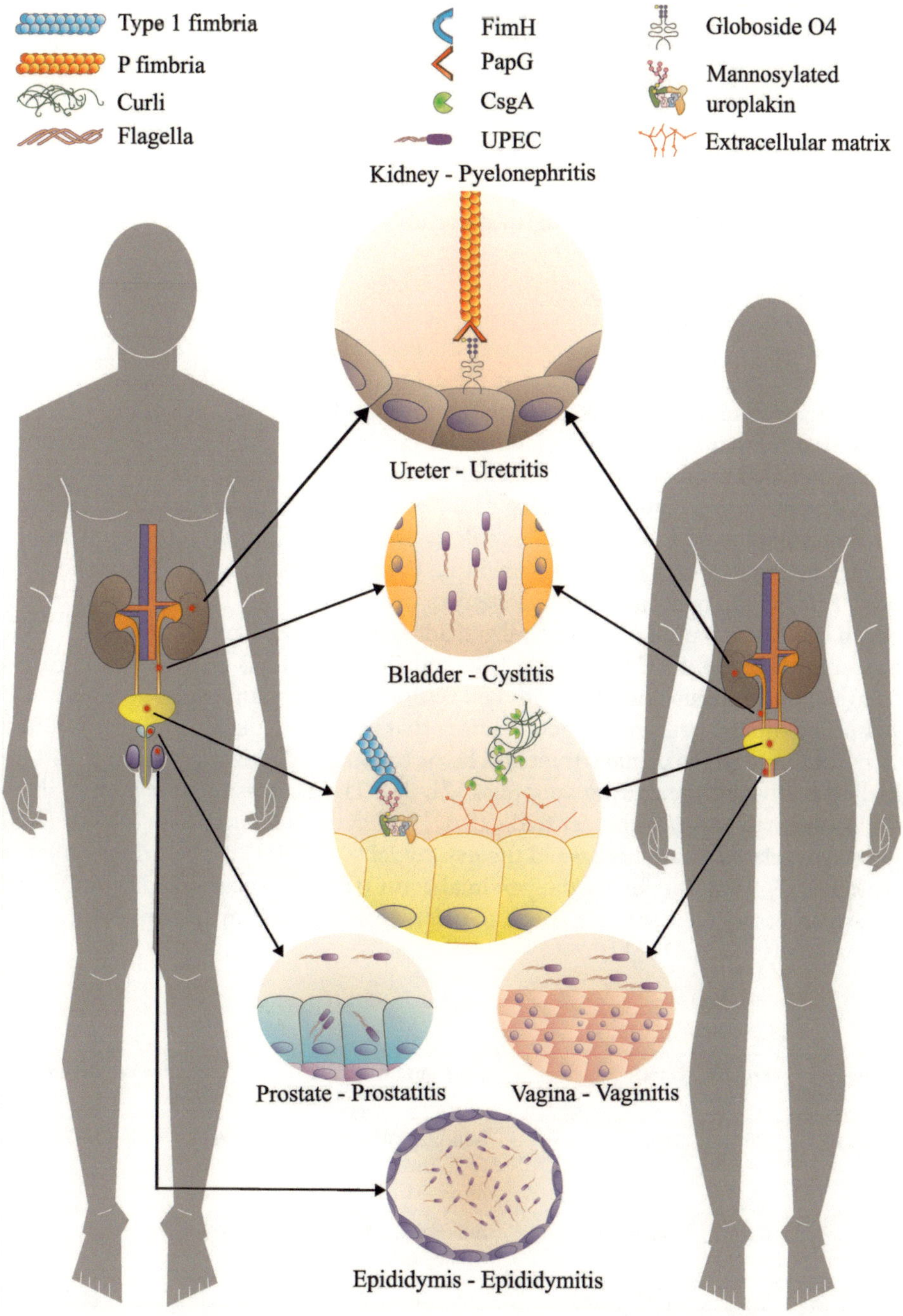

Figure 1.
Urinary tract infection localizations. Men and women have different localizations and usual reservoirs for complicated UTI. Infection establishment starts in the bladder by FimH adhesin from fimbria type 1 binding to mannosylated uroplakins, which are strongly associated with invasion processes, and by CsgA adhesin from Curli, which binds to the extracellular matrix. Some flagellated UPEC organisms are capable of ascending to the ureters and to the kidney; next, P fimbriae bind to globoside receptors by the recognition of PapG. In male patients, the forms of infection and probable reservoirs involve the prostate and epididymis. In the prostate, invasion of the epithelia has also been observed, while in the epididymis, metabolically active UPEC bacteria have been localized in the ducts. In female patients, the vagina is a reported reservoir. In the prostate, vagina, and epididymis, the adhesins involved in the adherence and invasive process are not known.

pathogenic *E. coli* (APEC), and mammary pathogenic *E. coli* (MPEC) [10]. Diarrheagenic *E. coli* strains and ExPEC have been recovered from animal infections, such as pneumonia in pigs, bovine and porcine mastitis, pyometra, and UTI in dogs [13, 14].

2. Virulence of UPEC to the urinary tract

UPEC is the leading etiological agent and has been related to more than 80% of UTIs [15]. The plasticity of this bacterium has allowed it to acquire different pathogenic attributes as tools to colonize the epithelium of the urinary tract. Analysis of various UPEC genomes has shown that the acquisition of virulence factors occurs in pathogenicity islands, plasmids, and phages through horizontal gene transfer [16]. Some virulence factors are secreted, while others are anchored in the outer membrane as molecules that promote bacterial colonization of the urinary tract and, therefore, the development of a clinical pathology [17]. Among the main colonization and virulence factors involved in UPEC pathogenicity are toxins, fimbriae, iron acquisition systems, autotransporter proteins, flagellum, lipopolysaccharides (LPS), and capsules [7, 18]. Briefly, the pathogenicity mechanism of UPEC mainly begins with adherence through the participation of three fimbrial adhesins (FimH, PapG, and CsgA), which are assembled in the distal part (type 1, P, and Curli fimbriae) as shown in **Figure 1** [19, 20]. These adhesins interact with cell receptors (α-D-mannosylated proteins, glycosphingolipids, neuraminic acid, factors that accelerate decay, and extracellular matrix proteins) in the urinary tract and favor bacterial colonization through different signaling pathways, generating apoptosis [21, 22]. The expression of α-hemolysin (HlyA), secreted autotransporter toxin (Sat), and cytotoxic necrotizing factor (CNF-1) has been related to an increase in the cytotoxicity of UPEC to the urinary tract (**Table 1**) [17]. Iron uptake *via* the yersiniabactin (*fyuA*) and aerobactin (*iutD*) systems are necessary elements for UPEC to colonize and persist in anatomical areas with low iron levels (**Table 1**) [17].

Category	Proteins	Name	Function	Evaluated in vaccines	Reference
Adhesin	FimH	Type 1 fimbriae	Adherence to the uroepithelium; binding to mannosylated residues	Yes	[7, 23–30]
	CsgA	Fimbriae P	Adherence to kidney cells; binding to sphingolipids	Yes	[7, 23]
	PapG	Curli	Adherence to the uroepithelium; binding to the extracellular matrix	Yes	[7, 23, 24, 27]
Hemolysin	HlyA	Alpha hemolysin	Increase in cytotoxic capabilities	Yes	[17, 23]
Toxin	Sat	Secreted autotransporter toxin	Increase in cytotoxic capabilities	No	[17]
	CNF-1	Cytotoxic necrotizing Factor	Increase in cytotoxic capabilities	No	[17]

Category	Proteins	Name	Function	Evaluated in vaccines	Reference
	Vat	Vacuolating autotransporter toxin	Increase in cytotoxic capabilities	No	[23]
Siderophore	FyuA	Yersiniabactin	Iron metabolism; iron acquisition	No	[17]
	IutA	Aerobactin	Iron metabolism; iron acquisition	Yes	[17, 29, 30]
	Ent	Enterobactin	Iron metabolism; iron acquisition	No	[23]
	IroN	Salmochelin receptor	Iron metabolism; iron acquisition	Yes	[23, 29, 30]
	ChuA	Heme receptor	Iron metabolism; iron acquisition	Yes	[29, 30]
	Hma	Haem acquisition protein	Iron metabolism; iron acquisition	Yes	[29, 30]
	Iha	Iron regulated-gene-homolog adhesin	Iron metabolism; iron acquisition	Yes	[29, 30]
	IreA	Catecholate siderophore (iron-regulating element)	Iron metabolism; iron acquisition	Yes	[29, 30]
Protectins	Iss	Increased Survival Serum factor	Bloodstream survival; critical for urosepsis development	No	[23]
	ProP	Proline permease	Osmoprotection; survival in urine	No	[31]
Motility	FliC	Flagella	Motility; related to pyelonephritis develop	Yes	[32]

Table 1.
UPEC virulence factors and their vaccine-evaluation status.

UPEC adhesion to the urinary tract cells is an initial process prior to the invasion, and a mechanism to withstand the flow of urine, the activity of antibodies and proteins with bactericidal properties, and the action of antibiotics (**Figure 2**) [33]. Invasion occurs through a "zipper" type mechanism, a process that involves the host cell membrane enveloping the bacteria *via* the activation of several proteins (tyrosine kinases, phosphoinositol-3 (PI-3) kinase, and cell division control proteins), which promote complexes between components of the cytoskeleton (actin, microtubules, and vinculin) [34]. Each of these steps allows UPEC to survive within macrophages as a mechanism of dissemination in the urinary tract [35]. In the cytoplasm, the bacterium initiates the formation of intracellular bacterial communities (IBCs) in three stages [early stage (IBC formation), intermediate stage (IBC maturation), and late stage (IBC efflux and release)], which are encapsulated in RAB27b spindle-shaped vesicles to associate with intermediate filaments of urinary tract cells (**Figure 2**) [36, 37]. The interaction of LPS with the "Toll"-like receptor (TLR) 4 favors an increase in cyclic adenosine monophosphate (cAMP) and the expulsion of UPEC wrapped in RAB27b^{+} vesicles [36, 38, 39]. TLR4 activation by UPEC *via* LPS, FimH, and/or PapG generates an intracellular oxidative state that causes filamentation by

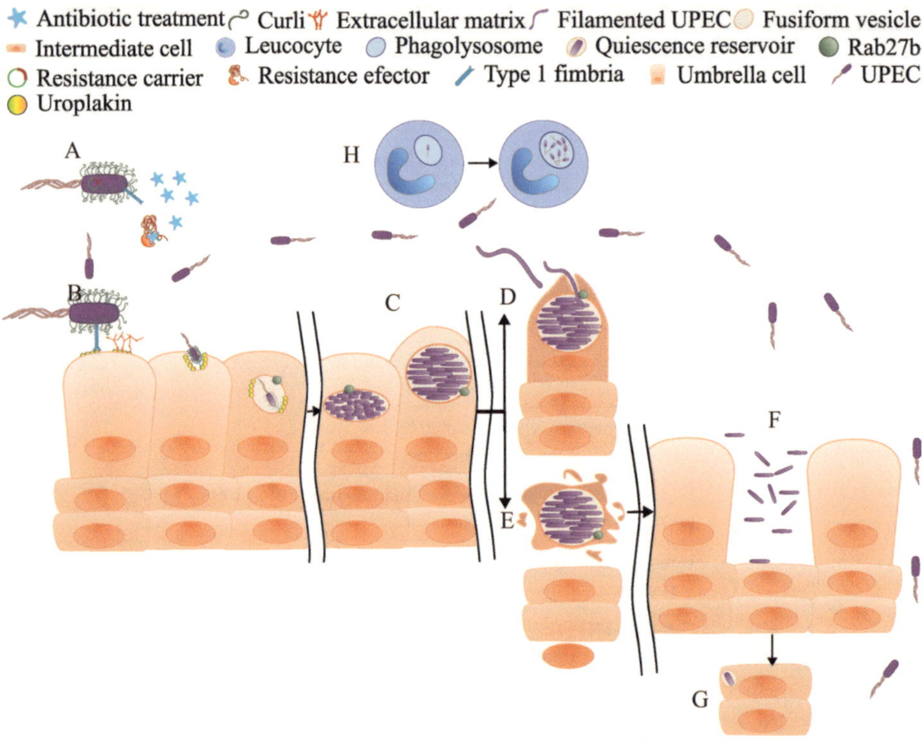

Figure 2.
Events associated with recurrence of urinary tract infections. A) Antibiotic resistance: UPEC strains can harbor resistance genes that allow them to evade the antibiotic function, with eventual failure of the antibiotic treatment. B) Adherence and invasion of UPEC: Fimbria type 1 binding facilitates invasion of the superficial cells from the uroepithelium, by the realigning of actin in Rab26b fusiform vesicles. Some of these vesicles can be released. C) Maturation of the intracellular bacterial community: After the invasion of cells by metabolically active UPEC strains, the bacteria multiply inside fusiform vesicles in a biofilm-like matrix. The increased stress environment makes division difficult, and the UPEC organisms appear as filiform nonsegmented bacteria. The maturation of this structure can lead to different paths. D) Efflux: Filiform bacteria can be released by the fusion of fusiform vesicles with the cellular membrane. E) Apoptosis: The host cell begins programmed cell death, and apoptosis results in the release of filiform bacteria. F) Adherence to intermediate cells: The apoptosis of superficial cells endangers the intermediate cells, and the UPEC bacteria bind to and invade this new layer. G) Quiescence reservoirs: In the intermediate cell layers, the UPEC organisms become quiescent, and these low-metabolic and nonmultiplying bacteria can lie dormant until a better environment is encountered, at which time the bacteria can readily reactivate. H) Strong resistance to phagocytosis: Some strains of UPEC are capable of resisting phagocytosis by neutrophils. By avoiding reactive oxygen species and resisting bactericidal mechanisms, UPEC organisms can be released from the phagolysosome.

inhibiting bacterial division [40]. The growth of UPEC filaments promotes host cell lysis, bacterial efflux, and the initiation of a new cycle of infection [41, 42]. Moreover, UPEC can enter a quiescent state for prolonged periods in exosomes, a mechanism that favors the bacteria to go unnoticed by the immune system (**Figure 2**) [43]. The TRP mucolipin-type channel 3 is expressed on the surface of exosomes activated by UPEC, promoting the neutralization and exocytosis of exosomes with bacteria in a quiescent state [44]. The release of UPEC wrapped in spindle-shaped vesicles is probably promoted by its fusion in the cell membrane of the uroepithelium, where the increase in the cell surface and distention of the bladder is favored (**Figure 2**) [45]. The exit of the bacteria from the quiescent state promotes the reinfection of the urinary tract by the same bacteria, defined as a recurrent UTI (RUTI), and its complications lead to the presence of pyelonephritis and urosepsis [45, 46]. UPEC pathogenicity, through different mechanisms, promotes colonization, persistence, and recurrence of infection, although the host also mounts an immune response against UTIs.

3. UPEC is mainly responsible for recurrent urinary tract infections (RUTIs)

UTIs are an inflammatory response to the colonization and multiplication of a microorganism, such as UPEC, mainly in any organ of the urinary system, which are accompanied by symptoms, such as dysuria, hematuria, urinary frequency and urgency, and occasionally suprapubic pain [47, 48]. UTIs occur more frequently in women, and the incidence rate of cystitis has been reported to be 12.6% in women and 3.0% in men in the USA [49]. Additionally, it has been estimated that 25% of UTI cases will present a new infectious episode after 3 months [50].

RUTIs occur when a patient has more than two episodes of UTIs within 6 months or more than three episodes within 1 year [51]. RUTIs represent a global health problem and have been related to poor clinical outcomes and a negative impact on patient's quality of life [52]. Recurrent cystitis in women and children is one of the most frequent infections; such episodes are usually disabling and present a more significant number of symptoms, and more than 80.3% are treated with various antibiotics. Recurrence prophylaxis is a clinical option; however, 73% of antibiotic prophylaxis patients have persistent infections and a high percentage have mental stress [53]. The incidence and prevalence of UTIs vary and depend on age, sex, and comorbidities. In Mexico, the epidemiological journal of the Ministry of Health recently reported 4,348,079 cases of UTIs, considering patients from <2 years to >60 years. UTIs are the third cause of morbidity in the Mexican population, with a higher-frequency age group between 25 and 44 years; however, in pediatric patients, UTIs are the most frequent infections considered healthcare-associated infections (HAIs). The rate of recurrence of UTIs in pediatrics is 15–20%, especially in the first year of life; after an initial case, the risk increases with the number of previous occurrences, ranging from 60 to 75% of cases with three or more occurrences [54, 55]. Timely diagnosis of RUTIs in pediatric patients is complicated since the signs and symptoms reported by the patient, or in some cases by family members, may be nonspecific. The damage that a RUTI can cause in this age group can be reflected in poor growth and anatomical function of the urinary tract, in addition to the generation of antimicrobial resistance in pediatric strains [55].

One of the essential characteristics of RUTIs is the number of previous infectious episodes, and it has been identified that when there is a history of previous episodes, the recurrence rate is 25% with an increase of up to 75% when there are more than two episodes [56]. Complications of UTIs can lead to changes in kidney function, even where the first episode of acute pyelonephritis can be the cause of kidney damage in 57% of cases [3, 57]. In children, one of the most critical risk factors for RUTI is urinary reflux, alone or in combination with dysfunctional urination [58, 59]. A second important risk factor is antimicrobial therapy since, in recent years, it has become more common to observe an increase in resistance to different antimicrobials in different parts of the world [60, 61]. This situation is complicated in children with vesical-urinary reflux because they require prophylactic treatment for prolonged periods, which invariably contributes to the selection of resistant strains.

Recently, RUTIs have been considered reinfections in the urinary tract; in these cases, it is considered that the etiological agent is usually different from the one that caused the initial symptoms. Among the associated microorganisms are *Klebsiella* spp., *Proteus* spp., and *Enterobacter* spp., and the participation of new and different strains of *E. coli*, a microorganism that in the RUTI is also considered the main agent responsible for this disease. Under this proposal, it has been proposed that the selective pressure exerted by antimicrobials during therapy is one of the factors responsible for the emergence of new strains of *E. coli* resistant to antimicrobials, considering the intestine as the main reservoir of the bacteria [62].

Generally, RUTIs are caused by different strains than those that caused the original condition; therefore, a RUTI is considered a reinfection with a new clinical strain [63]. Other studies have reported that in 50–78% of the cases, the collected strains contain the same characteristics as the identified initial strains; thus, the infection is considered a persistence of the original strain [64, 65]. The persistence of UPEC strains in the bladder could be related to their presence as part of the fecal biota for long periods, leading to recurrent ascending infections [4]. Local treatment of the perineum with antibiotics does not prevent the recurrence of UTIs, which indicates that the migration of the pathogen from the anus to the urinary tract is not an event associated with RUTIs (**Figure 2**) [66]. There are reservoirs of intracellular bacteria that persist for weeks and months in the urethral epithelium. Likewise, bacterial communities, as structures similar to biofilms, have been identified in the cells of women with cystitis. Other data have confirmed that UPEC strains invade the epithelium and form reservoirs of bacteria to produce RUTIs (**Figure 2**) [67–69]. In a study carried out from 2007 to 2011, the authors described 75 cases of RUTI whose etiological agent was UPEC strains; 52% (39/75) of them were persistent infections, and 48% (36/75) were associated with reinfections [63]. The average persistence fluctuated between 15 days and 42 months regarding reinfections. In addition, some patients presented reinfection by different UPEC strains for more than 36 months. This information reflects the importance of both clinical events (persistence and reinfection), with a high possibility of kidney damage due to the duration of the infectious process.

4. UPEC resistance impacts the course of UTI

Multidrug resistance (MDR) is a critical factor in UPEC strains that cause RUTIs worldwide due to the high costs of antimicrobial treatments [70]. One of the main resistance mechanisms is the participation of genes that code for extended-spectrum β-lactamases (ESBLs) and resistance genes that code for quinolones and sulfonamides [71]. Additionally, three mechanisms by which UPECr may cause RUTIs have been suggested: (1) The presence of resistance genes, which can cause treatment failure, as well as the selection of MDR strains that persist in the urinary tract. UPEC MDR strains can reactivate once treatment is completed. (2) The activation of invasins, toxins, siderophores, and metabolic fitness factors allows the invasion of uroepithelial cells, forming IBCs. In this process, the UPECr strains remain inside the cells of the transitional urinary epithelium, isolated and protected from antimicrobial treatment and the host's immune response. (3) The formation of quiescent reservoirs (QRs) by UPECr strains is maintained in the deepest layers of the urinary epithelium, where they can remain for long periods and be reactivated by various signaling systems that have not been described in detail (**Figure 2**). These mechanisms can be independent or act jointly in a single process. For the prevention of RUTIs, specifically in women, various treatment options, including continuous antibiotic prophylaxis, accompanied by behavioral therapy, probiotics, estrogens, and intravesical instillations of hyaluronate, have been proposed. However, the results have shown variable efficacy in the short and long term [72].

5. Use of antimicrobials in UTIs

The World Health Organization (WHO) has considered that the excessive use of antimicrobials is one of the main causes related to the increase in bacterial resistance, generating an important public health problem of inadequate medical prescription, excessive use, and increasingly (and sometimes unnecessarily) prolonged times in the treatment schemes. In addition, the administration of nonoptimal doses and failures in medication consumption has contributed significantly to the increase in antimicrobial resistance rates [73, 74]. The purpose of antimicrobial treatments against UTIs is to use antibiotics that guarantee the eradication of the responsible microorganisms, such as UPEC; however, it is crucial to consider the exact timing of antibiotic use to avoid adverse side effects. The selection of antimicrobials will depend on the causal agent, the sensitivity patterns in the community and/or hospital environment, and patient's characteristics (age, sex, pregnancy, anatomical location of the infection, and comorbid conditions). Factors related to the antimicrobial to be used include its pharmacodynamics, adverse effect profile, and ease of administration [75].

In general terms, antimicrobial therapy resolves most symptomatic cases of UTIs. Among the most frequently used antibiotics of choice are trimethoprim-sulfamethoxazole (TMP-SMX), fluoroquinolones, nitrofurantoin, amoxicillin with or without clavulanic acid, second- and third-generation cephalosporins, and aminoglycosides. In recent years, issues related to inadequate drug management, such as incomplete dosages, intolerance, and side effects, have been host factors that, together with bacterial resistance to antibiotics, lead to failures in the management and treatment of infections. In cases of complicated UTIs, the duration of antibiotic treatment should not be less than 7 days, and between 10 and 15 days is recommended. Severe infections often require treatment with broad-spectrum cephalosporins, such as cefotaxime or ceftriaxone, or with other beta-lactams that have excellent activity against microorganisms and good tissue penetration. A clinical study conducted in the United States of America (USA) showed that of 10,161 urine culture samples, 17% of *E. coli* and *P. mirabilis* isolates, 11% of *K. pneumoniae* isolates, and 3% of *Streptococcus saprophyticus* isolates were resistant to TMP-SMX. However, the frequencies and antimicrobials vary between hospital-acquired and community-acquired infections; an example is resistance to ampicillin (63%) in *E. coli* isolates from samples of nonhospitalized children in Israel.

Recently, in the HIMFG, we described some specific characteristics of 105 UPEC strains isolated from urine samples of children diagnosed with acute UTIs, observing a resistance rate of 86% for ampicillin, 69% for amoxicillin-clavulanic acid, and 55% for nalidixic acid. Regarding the presence of multidrug resistance, 19% of the isolates were resistant to 3 or more groups of antibiotics. In 2010, a prospective study of UTIs, including 289 *E. coli,* isolates showed that 78% were resistant to ampicillin; 60%, to trimethoprim-sulfamethoxazole; 40%, to ciprofloxacin; 50%, to ceftriaxone; and 32%, to gentamicin. These data show how resistance to the different antimicrobials used for treating UTIs is maintained with a high frequency and, in some cases, higher than that reported in other parts of the world.

6. Biofilms formed by UPEC favor the development of UTIs

The formation of biofilms by UPEC is a process that is made up of a series of sequential events, where virulence and aptitude factors are activated and repressed; in addition, it is regulated by environmental signals that allow the change in the condition of planktonic cells until the establishment of biofilms, with the relevant changes in the gene expression of bacterial strains [76, 77]. Bacteria express various virulent factors through the use of nutrients to form biofilms, which change their spatial organization and alter the expression of surface molecules as a mechanism of resistance to environmental stress. Changes in environmental conditions within the bacterial biofilm can lead to the emergence of bacterial subpopulations that express different genes in response to the availability of nutrients and oxygen [78–80]. Biofilms, as highly organized structures, confer an advantage to bacterial pathogenesis and make eradicating such organisms more complex, resulting in chronic infection. Biofilm formation during UTIs is an event that can lead to severe infections in hospitalized and community patients [81, 82]. UPEC is the uropathogen most closely related to RUTIs, employing a complex pathogenic cascade to colonize extra- and intracellular niches during the infectious process [83]. UPEC strains activate numerous virulence factors during colonization of the urinary tract, such as adhesins, toxins, iron acquisition systems, capsular structures, flagellum, and islands of pathogenicity [82, 84, 85]. The processes of adhesion, invasion, and formation of CBI as mechanisms that contribute to the persistence of UPEC are related to the expression of external appendages, known as fimbriae or pili (**Figure 2**). Several fimbriae that participate in the adherence to various epithelia (such as the urothelium) or processes of invasion and CBI formation, thereby facilitating the persistence of UPEC, have been described (**Figure 2**).

Bacterial biofilms are a significant cause of antibiotic resistance and infection persistence; in this context, biofilm control is essential in reducing MDR bacterial infections. Recently, the reuse of drugs with anti-biofilm activity has been implemented in treating UTIs due to UPEC. Auranofin is a drug approved by the FDA in 1985 for treating rheumatoid arthritis and has shown effectiveness as an antibacterial agent [86]. Interestingly, auranofin significantly inhibits the biofilm formation of UPEC strains [87]. Likewise, trans-cinnamaldehyde (CNMA) is a natural molecule derived from *Cinnamomum zeylanicum*, which has shown its usefulness in treating high blood pressure and low blood glucose in diabetic patients. CNMA and its derivatives maintain an antimicrobial spectrum and anti-biofilm activity against UPEC at a minimum inhibitory concentration of 50–100 μg/mL. Additionally, they inhibit flagellar mobility and reduce the production of extracellular polymeric substances in UPEC [88]. Trans-resveratrol and oxyresveratrol are compounds with antimicrobial, antiviral, antioxidant, anti-inflammatory, anticancer, neuroprotective, and anti-biofilm activities against several bacterial pathogens [89–93].

Trans-resveratrol and oxyresveratrol significantly reduce biofilm formation by UPEC at sub-inhibitory concentrations of 10–50 μg/mL, and they also present an antivirulence strategy against the persistence of bacterial infections through a reduction in the production of fimbriae and swarming mobility. Furthermore, t-resveratrol and oxiresveratrol markedly decrease the hemagglutinating capacity of UPEC and increase the killing of bacteria by the human blood complex [94]. Finally, many plant-derived compounds can act in conjunction with existing antibiotics. A synergistic effect has been demonstrated between Type A procyanidin and the antibiotic nitrofurantoin at pH 5.8 due to a deregulation process of the expression of UPEC fimbrial adhesins [95]. These studies support the need to carry out synergism tests between various agents used in treating chronic diseases and derived from plants in conjunction with antibiotics as a strategy to identify anti-biofilm agents and with antimicrobial effects that support the treatment of infections by UPEC-MDR [87].

7. Fimbria type 1, PapG, and Curli in the CBI process by UPEC

UPEC is the main uropathogen recovered in more than 80% of RUTIs [96]. The pathophysiology of RUTIs due to UPEC is a complex process that has not yet been fully characterized. Several studies have described the participation of various virulence factors associated with UPEC pathogenicity, such as adhesion fimbriae: *fim* (fimbria type 1), *csg* (Curli), *pap* (fimbria P); siderophores: *ent* (enterobactin), *iut* (aerobactin), *fyu* (yersiniabactin); toxins: *hly* (hemolysin), sat (autotransporter secreted toxin), vat (autotransporter vacuolating toxin); and capsule production and variations in lipopolysaccharides. The presence of metabolic regulators and protectins, such as *iss* (factor for increasing serum survival) and *pro* (proline permease), also have an essential role in the persistence of UPEC (**Table 1**) [23].

8. Nonantibiotic alternatives for the treatment of UTIs

The vaccines available for treating of UTIs are products focused on stimulating the systemic immune response due to the difficulty of stimulating mucosal immunity [97]. Different bacterial antigens, such as O antigen (major compound of LPS), FimCH (bound of the FimC chaperone and FimH adhesin), and PapDG (the bound to the chaperone PapD and PapG adhesin), HlyA and IroN, have generated a systemic specific response but not generated a response at the mucosa level (**Table 1**) [24–27]. Indeed, bacterial antigens efficiently induce mucosal immunogenicity *via* intranasal (IN), intravaginal, and oral administration. Meanwhile, parenteral administration induces an inefficient response [98].

The SolcoUrovac® vaccine approach (rebranded StroVac®) is a formulation from a suspension of 10 *E. coli*, which were inactivated from different serotypes and including other uropathogens. Administration through the vaginal mucosa significantly reduces recurrent UTIs, according to phase II clinical studies; however, they have generated adverse reactions such as pain and irritation of the vaginal epithelium (**Table 2**) [99, 100]. In a randomized, double-binding, placebo-controlled, parallel-group study, intramuscular administration of three injections 2 weeks apart showed a nonstatistical reduction in clinically relevant UTI episodes (86/188 patients, 46.0%) when compared with the placebo group (97/188 patients, 51.6%). However, the same data showed a statistical reduction of UTIs in patients with more than seven UTIs in the previous year [101].

The oral administration of the immunomodulator Urostim®, another uropathogens lysate, in phase clinical II the one tablet dose for 3 months, stimulates the cellular phagocytosis and secretory IgA humoral response, without generating protection against UTIs [31]. Oral administration of OM-89/Uro-Vaxom®, a lyophilizate biological extract from 18 *E. coli* strains, reduces RUTIs; however, it produces adverse effects related to immunological tolerance and clinical manifestations at the gastrointestinal level (**Table 2**) [102].

Name	Formulation	Administration	Doses and treatment duration	Adverse responses and protection effect
SolcoUrovac® vaccine (rebranded StroVac®)	Heat lysate of 10 uropathogenic strains, *Escherichia coli* (6), *Morganella morganii*, *Proteus mirabilis*, *Enterococcus faecalis* and *Klebsiella pneumoniae*.	Intramuscular injection	Three injections of 0.5 mL, at intervals from 1 to 2 weeks.	Significant reduction in RUTI. There are no long-term clinical studies. Localized adverse reactions such as pain and irritation. Systemic reactions such as fever, headache, dizziness, and nausea.
Immunomodulator Urostim®	Uropathogenic bacterial lysates from *E. coli*, *P. mirabilis*, *E. faecalis*, and *K. pneumoniae*	Oral	One tablet per day for two to three consecutive months.	Stimulation of the cellular and humoral response. It does not generate protection.
OM-89/Uro-Vaxom® vaccine	Lyophilized biological extract of *E. coli* (18c).	Oral	One tablet per day for three consecutive months.	Reduction in recurring UTIs. It produces immunological tolerance and clinical manifestations at the gastrointestinal level, diarrhea, nausea, and abdominal pain. At the cutaneous level, it can lead to pruritus and rash.
ExPEC4V vaccine	Conjugated with the exotoxin A of *Pseudomonas aeruginosa* bound to four polysaccharide antigens of the serotypes of *E. coli* O1A, O2, O6A, and O25B.	Intramuscular	One intramuscular injection of 0.5 mL.	Low reduction in RUTIs; mild adverse effects.
UROMUNE® (MV140) vaccine	Whole bacterial cells from inactive uropathogens: *E. coli*, *Proteus vulgaris*, *E. faecalis*, and *K. pneumoniae*	Sublingual	Two sprays daily for 3 to 6 months.	Reduction of 55.7% and 58% in the frequency of RUTIs in 3 and 6 months of treatment, respectively. The 1.7% of patients manifest mild adverse effects.

Table 2.
Available commercial vaccines for the treatment and prevention of RUTI.

The ExPEC4V conjugate vaccine is a long-term development for a bioconjugate of exotoxin A from *P. aeruginosa* with four polysaccharide antigens of *E. coli* strains. The parental vaccination with the tetravalent o-conjugate was well tolerated with mild adverse events but safe. A preliminary study showed a low UTI reduction; the functional immune response was shown for a bacterial count reduction (**Table 2**) [103, 104]. The efficacy and safety of the UROMUNE® (MV140) vaccine showed only 1.7% of mild adverse responses. This vaccine was generated with glycerinated suspensions of heat-inactivated whole bacteria of four uropathogens and administrated daily by a sublingual spray for 3 months. While reported evidence suggests that this vaccine can be effective, reports concluded that some patients with RUTI can achieve a non-UTI status (**Table 2**) [105].

Finally, the transurethral immunization of mice with attenuated UPEC strains is not persistent in the urinary tract and favors nonspecific protection [106]. Intranasal immunization (IN) with different UPEC antigens (ChuA, Hma, Iha, IreA, IroN, IutA, and FimH) induces the activation of high concentrations of IgA in saliva, vagina, and urine (**Table 1**) [29, 30]. According to this information, IN vaccination of fimbrial adhesins may be a potential strategy to generate a humoral immune response with IgA antibodies in the mucosa of the urinary tract as a mechanism of host protection against UTIs by UPEC.

9. Fimbrial adhesins and immune response

Various studies have described the development of effective strategies for the prevention, treatment, and/or management of UTIs caused by UPEC. However, there are no effective vaccines generated from fimbrial adhesins, autotransporters, toxins, siderophores, flagella, and outer membrane proteins of UPEC. These proteins, located on the bacterial surface, are expressed during infectious processes and can stimulate an immune response from the host [107]. UPEC mainly expresses three types of fimbrial adhesins during the colonization of urinary tract cells: FimH located in the upper part of the type 1 fimbria, PapG in the P fimbria, and CsgA in the Curli fimbriae [19].

Data generated by our working group have revealed that 90% of clinical strains of UPEC isolated from pediatric patients express fimbria type 1. This fimbrial adhesin has been related to adherence, invasion, and formation of bacterial colonies in the urinary tract (**Figure 2**) [108]. In addition, we have reported that more than 95% of clinical strains of UPEC contain csgA, a gene that codes for the CsgA protein (a structural adhesin of the Curli fimbriae) and has been associated with urosepsis processes [109, 110]. More than 35% of UPEC clinical strains express the P fimbria, a homopolymeric structure that participates in the colonization of the kidney *via* interaction with globoceramides located in renal cells. The diversity of globoceramides in the kidney has favored the appearance of three allelic variants in the papG gene [papGJ96 (variant I), papGAD/IA2 (variant II), and prsGJ96 (variant III)] [111]. It is important to note that the FimH, CsgA, and PapGII adhesins are three essential protein structures in the pathogenesis of UPEC and may be viable biomolecules for the generation of an effective vaccine that stimulates an immune response.

10. FimH of type 1 fimbria is immunogenic

The FimH adhesin (fimbria type 1) is a protein used in preliminary studies in animal models to evaluate its potential as a viable vaccine. Sera from C3H/HeJ mice immunized with the FimH adhesin and type 1 fimbria inhibit adherence to human bladder cells [28]. Other studies have shown that the mannose-binding domain of FimH, plus the complete protein and in association with FimC (flagellin and chaperone), significantly reduces adherence in the bladder and kidney in mice and cynomolgus monkeys; in addition, specific anti-FimH antibodies inhibit the colonization of UPEC [26, 28, 112–114]. The recombinant FimH protein fused with the FliC protein induces a significant increase in the cellular and humoral immune response against UTIs in a murine model [101]. Subcutaneous immunization induced high levels of immunoglobulins (IgG1 and IgG2a) and cytokines [(INFγ: interferon gamma) and IL4 (interleukin 4)] [32]. IN immunization with FimH (UPEC) and MrpH (*P. mirabilis*) protein as a fused molecule induces the release of IgG and IgA antibodies in mouse samples (serum, urine, nasal wash, and vaginal). Th1- and Th2-type cellular immunity generated by FimH/MrpH proteins with or without MPL adjuvant suggests that one of these proteins functions as an adjuvant molecule [115]. The FimH protein interacts with TLR4 through the α-mannosylated coreceptor, favoring the activation of CD4- epithelial cells *via* Tirap-MyD88 to recruit neutrophils in the mucosa [116, 117].

11. The PapG adhesin is an immunogenic molecule

The expression of the adhesin PapG contributes to the UPEC colonization in the kidney during the pyelonephritis process in humans [118]. The interaction of PapG with TLR4 activates the secretion of IL-6 and IL-8 [118, 119]. Intraperitoneal immunization of the P fimbria and a protein complex of PapDG (chaperone) generates protection against kidney inflammation and production induces specific antibodies in mice and cynomolgus monkey sera [24, 120]. In these studies, no significant differences showed between the number of bacteria recovered in urine and the control group, probably due to the expression of other accessory fimbriae involved in bacterial colonization [81].

12. CsgA is an immunogenic protein

Preliminary data obtained by our working group showed that CsgA from the Curli fimbriae is an adhesin that contributes as an accessory molecule in the adherence of UPEC to bladder cells; however, more studies are still required to determine the specific role in the pathogenesis of UPEC [110]. High levels of anti-CsgA antibodies recognize the CsgA protein in sera from patients convalescing from sepsis. These data suggest the expression of the protein *in vivo*; however, more studies are necessary to evaluate the immunogenicity of this protein [110]. In other *E. coli*, the Curli fimbriae induce the release of proinflammatory cytokines (TNFα, IL6, and IL8) in macrophage cells [121]. The recombinant protein CsgA from *Salmonella* and Curli from *E. coli* MC4100 participate in the release of IL8 in human THP-1 macrophage cells through the cooperative interaction of TLR1 and TLR2 [122]. The CsgA protein has also been considered a pathogen-associated molecular pattern (PAMP), responsible for generating an IL6 and IL1β response *via* the inflammasome (NLRP3) [123, 124].

13. Conclusions

Several studies have reported that UPEC is responsible for 90% of community UTIs and approximately 60% of hospital-acquired UTIs; however, more studies are required to elucidate the specific characteristics of UPEC, such as its serotypes, virulence factors, and antimicrobial susceptibility. The innate plasticity of the genome of this bacterium allows it to acquire various virulence factors, resistance mechanisms, and adaptative advantages to colonize the urinary tract. The presence of clinical strains of MDR and XDR UPEC is a highly worrisome phenomenon that alerts health specialists who are left without therapeutic options to treat acute and recurrent UTIs effectively. The FimH, CsgA, and PapG adhesins are the main virulence factors of UPEC. These adhesins can be considered new targets in the elaboration of biomolecules with immunogenic potential for protection against UTIs.

The search for new alternative antibiotics has led to the emergence of potential biomolecules that can generate an efficient vaccine that protects against UTIs, significantly reducing or eliminating disease cases. These biomolecules with the capacity to generate protection can act alone or in association with antibiotics of a lesser spectrum for treating UTIs. Recently, we reported that the best way to generate protection is by intranasal inoculation of mixtures of these protein adhesins with the ability to generate antibodies in mucous membranes; however, more studies are still necessary to solidify this premise. Finally, frontier science may lead us to the paradigm of improving our understanding of mucosal immunity and the role of these adhesin-based biomolecules as an alternative to the overuse of antimicrobials to treat UTIs.

Acknowledgements

The data generated by my workgroup and published in other journals have been approached in this book chapter with an integral focus on addressing their relevance to UTIs. The different experiments conducted were supported by Public Federal Funds HIM-2017-107 SSA. 1421, HIM-2018-045 SSA. 1503, HIM-2019-038 SSA. 1592, and HIM-2021-030 FF SSA. 1730 from the Hospital Infantil de México Federico Gómez. These grants were approved by the Research Committee (Dr. Juan Garduño Espinosa), Ethics Committee (Dr. Luis Jasso Gutiérrez), and Biosecurity Committee (Dr. Marcela Salazar García) of Hospital Infantil de México Federico Gómez.

Conflict of interest

The authors declare no conflict of interest.

Abbreviations

UPEC	uropathogenic *E. coli*
UTI	urinary tract infection
RUTI	recurrent urinary tract infections
MDR	multidrug-resistant
XDR	extensively drug-resistant
CFU	colony-forming units
IBCs	intracellular bacterial communities
LPS	lipopolysaccharides
TLR	"Toll"-like receptor
cAMP	cyclic adenosine monophosphate
TRP	transient receptor potential
HAIs	healthcare-associated infections

ESBL	extended-spectrum β-lactamases
UPECr	UPEC recurrent strains
QR	quiescent reservoirs
WHO	World Health Organization
IN	intranasal immunization
MPL®	monophosphoryl lipid A
IL	interleukin
PAMP	pathogen-associated molecular patterns
TNFα	tumor necrosis factor-alpha
NLRP3	NOD-, LRR- and pyrin domain-containing protein

Author details

Juan Xicohtencatl-Cortes[1]*, Sara A. Ochoa[1], Ariadnna Cruz-Córdova[1], Marco A. Flores-Oropeza[1] and Rigoberto Hernández-Castro[2]

1 Laboratorio de Investigación en Bacteriología Intestinal, Hospital Infantil de México Federico Gómez, Ciudad de México, Mexico

2 Departamento de Ecología de Agentes Patógenos, Hospital General "Dr. Manuel Gea González", Ciudad de México, Mexico

*Address all correspondence to: juanxico@yahoo.com

References

[1] Jacobsen SM, Stickler DJ, Mobley HL, Shirtliff ME. Complicated catheter-associated urinary tract infections due to *Escherichia coli* and *Proteus mirabilis*. Clinical Microbiology Reviews. 2008;**21**: 26-59. DOI: 10.1128/cmr.00019-07

[2] Beetz R, Mannhardt W, Fisch M, Stein R, Thüroff JW. Long-term follow-up of 158 young adults surgically treated for vesicoureteral reflux in childhood: The ongoing risk of urinary tract infections. The Journal of Urology. 2002; **168**:704-707; discussion 707. DOI: 10.1016/s0022-5347(05)64729-5

[3] Lin KY, Chiu NT, Chen MJ, Lai CH, Huang JJ, Wang YT, et al. Acute pyelonephritis and sequelae of renal scar in pediatric first febrile urinary tract infection. Pediatric Nephrology. 2003; **18**:362-365. DOI: 10.1007/s00467-003-1109-1

[4] Hooton TM. Clinical practice. Uncomplicated urinary tract infection. The New England Journal of Medicine. 2012;**366**:1028-1037. DOI: 10.1056/NEJMcp1104429

[5] Wilson ML, Gaido L. Laboratory diagnosis of urinary tract infections in adult patients. Clinical Infectious Diseases. 2004;**38**:1150-1158. DOI: 10.1086/383029

[6] Flores-Mireles AL, Walker JN, Caparon M, Hultgren SJ. Urinary tract infections: Epidemiology, mechanisms of infection and treatment options. Nature Reviews. Microbiology. 2015;**13**(5): 269-284. DOI: 10.1038/nrmicro3432

[7] Luna-Pineda VM, Ochoa S, Cruz-Córdova A, Cázares-Domínguez V, Vélez-González F, Hernández-Castro R, et al. Urinary tract infections, immunity, and vaccination. Boletin Medico del Hospital Infantil de Mexico. 2018;**75**: 67-78. DOI: 10.24875/bmhim.m18000011

[8] Levine MM. *Escherichia coli* that cause diarrhea: Enterotoxigenic, enteropathogenic, enteroinvasive, enterohemorrhagic, and enteroadherent. The Journal of Infectious Diseases. 1987; **155**(3):377-389. DOI: 10.1093/infdis/155.3.377

[9] Gomes TA, Elias WP, Scaletsky IC, Guth BE, Rodrigues JF, Piazza RM, et al. Diarrheagenic *Escherichia coli*. Brazilian Journal of Microbiology. 2016;**47**(Suppl 1):3-30. DOI: 10.1016/j.bjm.2016.10.015

[10] Sora VM, Meroni G, Martino PA, Soggiu A, Bonizzi L, Zecconi A. Extraintestinal pathogenic *Escherichia coli*: Virulence factors and antibiotic resistance. Pathogens. 2021;**10**(11):1355. DOI: 10.3390/pathogens10111355

[11] Foxman B, Brown P. Epidemiology of urinary tract infections: Transmission and risk factors, incidence, and costs. Infectious Disease Clinics of North America. 2003;**17**:227-241. DOI: 10.1016/S0891-5520(03)00005-9

[12] Riley LW. Pandemic lineages of Extraintestinal pathogenic *Escherichia coli*. Clinical Microbiology and Infection. 2014;**20**:380-390. DOI: 10.1111/1469-0691.12646

[13] Müştak HK, Günaydin E, Kaya İB, Salar MÖ, Babacan O, Önat K, et al. Phylo-typing of clinical *Escherichia coli* isolates originating from bovine mastitis and canine pyometra and urinary tract infection by means of quadruplex PCR. Veterinary Quarterly. 2015;**35**(4): 194-199. DOI: 10.1080/01652176.2015.1068963

[14] Kong L-C, Guo X, Wang Z, Gao Y-H, Jia B-Y, Liu S-M, et al. Whole genome sequencing of an ExPEC that caused fatal pneumonia at a pig farm in Changchun, China. BMC Veterinary Research. 2017;**13**:169. DOI: 10.1186/s12917-017-1093-5

[15] Kline KA, Lewis AL. Gram-positive uropathogens, polymicrobial urinary tract infection, and the emerging microbiota of the urinary tract. In: Mulvey MA, Klumpp DJ, Stapleton AE, editors. Urinary Tract Infections: Molecular Pathogenesis and Clinical Management. Chichester: Wiley; 2017. pp. 459-502

[16] Lloyd AL, Rasko DA, Mobley HL. Defining genomic islands and uropathogen-specific genes in uropathogenic *Escherichia coli*. Journal of Bacteriology. 2007;**189**:3532-3546. DOI: 10.1128/jb.01744-06

[17] Subashchandrabose S, Mobley HL. Virulence and fitness determinants of uropathogenic *Escherichia coli*. In: Mulvey MA, Klumpp DJ, Stapleton AE, editors. Urinary Tract Infections: Molecular Pathogenesis and Clinical Management. 2nd edition. Wiley; 2017. pp. 235-261. DOI: 10.1128/9781555817404.ch12

[18] Nielubowicz GR, Mobley HLT. Host–pathogen interactions in urinary tract infection. Nature Reviews Urology. 2010;**7**:430-441. DOI: 10.1038/nrurol.2010.101

[19] Antão E-M, Wieler LH, Ewers C. Adhesive threads of extraintestinal pathogenic *Escherichia coli*. Gut Pathogens. 2009;**1**:22. DOI: 10.1186/1757-4749-1-22

[20] Spaulding CN, Hultgren SJ. Adhesive pili in UTI pathogenesis and drug development. Pathogens. 2016;**5**: 30. DOI: 10.3390/pathogens5010030

[21] Lüthje P, Brauner A. Virulence factors of uropathogenic *E. coli* and their interaction with the host. Advances in Microbial Physiology. 2014;**65**:337-372. DOI: 10.1016/bs.ampbs.2014.08.006

[22] Thumbikat P, Berry RE, Zhou G, Billips BK, Yaggie RE, Zaichuk T, et al. Bacteria-induced uroplakin signaling mediates bladder response to infection. PLoS Pathogens. 2009;**5**:e1000415. DOI: 10.1371/journal.ppat.1000415

[23] Johnson JR, Russo TA. Acute pyelonephritis in adults. The New England Journal of Medicine. 2018;**378**: 48-59. DOI: 10.1056/nejmcp1702758

[24] Roberts JA, Kaack MB, Baskin G, Chapman MR, Hunstad DA, Pinkner JS, et al. Antibody responses and protection from pyelonephritis following vaccination with purified *Escherichia coli* PAPDG protein. The Journal of Urology. 2004;**171**:1682-1685. DOI: 10.1097/01.ju.0000116123.05160.43

[25] Russo TA, McFadden CD, Carlino-MacDonald UB, Beanan JM, Olson R, Wilding GE. The Siderophore receptor IroN of extraintestinal pathogenic *Escherichia coli* is a potential vaccine candidate. Infection and Immunity. 2003;**71**:7164-7169. DOI: 10.1128/iai.71.12.7164-7169.2003

[26] Langermann S, Möllby R, Burlein JE, Palaszynski SR, Auguste CG, DeFusco A, et al. Vaccination with FimH adhesin protects cynomolgus monkeys from colonization and infection by uropathogenic *Escherichia coli*. The Journal of Infectious Diseases. 2000;**181**: 774-778. DOI: 10.1086/315258

[27] O'Hanley P, Lalonde G, Ji G. Alpha-hemolysin contributes to the pathogenicity of piliated digalactoside-binding *Escherichia coli* in the kidney: Efficacy of an alpha-hemolysin vaccine

in preventing renal injury in the BALB/c mouse model of pyelonephritis. Infection and Immunity. 1991;**59**: 1153-1161. DOI: 10.1128/iai.59.3.1153-1161.1991

[28] Langermann S, Palaszynski S, Barnhart M, Auguste G, Pinkner JS, Burlein J, et al. Prevention of mucosal *Escherichia coli* infection by FimH-adhesin-based systemic vaccination. Science. 1997;**276**:607-611. DOI: 10.1126/science.276.5312.607

[29] Mike LA, Smith SN, Sumner CA, Eaton KA, Mobley HL. Siderophore vaccine conjugates protect against uropathogenic *Escherichia coli* urinary tract infection. Proceedings of the National Academy of Sciences of the United States of America. 2016;**113**: 13468-13473. DOI: 10.1073/pnas.1606324113

[30] Alteri CJ, Hagan EC, Sivick KE, Smith SN, Mobley HL. Mucosal immunization with iron receptor antigens protects against urinary tract infection. PLoS Pathogens. 2009;**5**: e1000586. DOI: 10.1371/journal.ppat.1000586

[31] Markova R, Nikolaeva S, Kostadinova R, Mitov I, et al. Cellular and humoral systemic and mucosal immune responses stimulated by an oral polybacterial immunomodulator in patients with chronic urinary tract infections. International Journal of Immunopathology and Pharmacology. 2005;**18**:457-473. DOI: 10.1177/039463200501800306

[32] Karam MRA, Oloomi M, Mahdavi M, Habibi M, Bouzari S. Vaccination with recombinant FimH fused with flagellin enhances cellular and humoral immunity against urinary tract infection in mice. Vaccine. 2013;**31**:1210-1216. DOI: 10.1016/j.vaccine.2012.12.059

[33] Dhakal BK, Kulesus RR, Mulvey MA. Mechanisms and consequences of bladder cell invasion by uropathogenic *Escherichia coli*. European Journal of Clinical Investigation. 2008;**38**(Suppl 2): 2-11. DOI: 10.1111/j.1365-2362.2008.01986.x

[34] Dhakal BK, Mulvey MA. Uropathogenic *Escherichia coli* invades host cells via an HDAC6-modulated microtubule-dependent pathway. The Journal of Biological Chemistry. 2009; **284**:446-454. DOI: 10.1074/jbc.M805010200

[35] Bokil NJ, Totsika M, Carey AJ, Stacey KJ, Hancock V, Saunders BM, et al. Intramacrophage survival of uropathogenic *Escherichia coli*: Differences between diverse clinical isolates and between mouse and human macrophages. Immunobiology. 2011;**216**:1164-1171. DOI: 10.1016/j.imbio.2011.05.011

[36] Bishop BL, Duncan MJ, Song J, Li G, Zaas D, Abraham SN. Cyclic AMP–regulated exocytosis of *Escherichia coli* from infected bladder epithelial cells. Nature Medicine. 2007;**13**:625-630. DOI: 10.1038/nm1572

[37] Scott VC, Haake DA, Churchill BM, Justice SS, Kim JH. Intracellular bacterial communities: A potential etiology for chronic lower urinary tract symptoms. Urology. 2015;**86**:425-431. DOI: 10.1016/j.urology.2015.04.002

[38] Song J, Bishop BL, Li G, Grady R, Stapleton A, Abraham SN. TLR4-mediated expulsion of bacteria from infected bladder epithelial cells. Proceedings of the National Academy of Sciences of the United States of America. 2009;**106**:14966-14971. DOI: 10.1073/pnas.0900527106

[39] Song J, Bishop BL, Li G, Duncan MJ, Abraham SN. TLR4-initiated and cAMP-

mediated abrogation of bacterial invasion of the bladder. Cell Host & Microbe. 2007;**1**:287-298. DOI: 10.1016/j.chom.2007.05.007

[40] Justice SS, Lauer SR, Hultgren SJ, Hunstad DA. Maturation of intracellular *Escherichia coli* communities requires SurA. Infection and Immunity. 2006;**74**:4793-4800. DOI: 10.1128/iai.00355-06

[41] Mulvey MA, Schilling JD, Martinez JJ, Hultgren SJ. Bad bugs and beleaguered bladders: Interplay between uropathogenic *Escherichia coli* and innate host defenses. Proceedings of the National Academy of Sciences of the United States of America. 2000;**97**:8829-8835. DOI: 10.1073/pnas.97.16.8829

[42] Klein K, Palarasah Y, Kolmos HJ, Møller-Jensen J, Andersen TE. Quantification of filamentation by uropathogenic *Escherichia coli* during experimental bladder cell infection by using semi-automated image analysis. Journal of Microbiological Methods. 2015;**109**:110-116. DOI: 10.1016/j.mimet.2014.12.017

[43] Leatham-Jensen MP, Mokszycki ME, Rowley DC, Deering R, Camberg JL, Sokurenko EV, et al. Uropathogenic *Escherichia coli* metabolite-dependent quiescence and persistence may explain antibiotic tolerance during urinary tract infection. mSphere. 2016;**1**:e00055-e00015. DOI: 10.1128/mSphere.00055-15

[44] Miao Y, Li G, Zhang X, Xu H, Abraham SN. A TRP channel senses lysosome neutralization by pathogens to trigger their expulsion. Cell. 2015;**161**:1306-1319. DOI: 10.1016/j.cell.2015.05.009

[45] Truschel ST, Wang E, Ruiz WG, Leung SM, Rojas R, Lavelle J, et al. Stretch-regulated exocytosis/endocytosis in bladder umbrella cells. Molecular Biology of the Cell. 2002;**13**:830-846. DOI: 10.1091/mbc.01-09-0435

[46] Kodner CM, Thomas Gupton EK. Recurrent urinary tract infections in women: Diagnosis and management. American Family Physician. 2010;**82**:638-643

[47] Anger J, Lee U, Ackerman AL, Chou R, Chughtai B, Clemens JQ, et al. Recurrent uncomplicated urinary tract infections in women: AUA/CUA/SUFU guideline. Journal of Urology. 2019;**202**:282-289. DOI: 10.1097/JU.0000000000000296

[48] Burnett LA, Hochstedler BR, Weldon K, Wolfe AJ, Brubaker L. Recurrent urinary tract infection: Association of clinical profiles with urobiome composition in women. Neurourology and Urodynamics. 2021;**40**:1479-1489. DOI: 10.1002/nau.24707

[49] Wagenlehner FME, Bjorklund Johansen TE, Cai T, Koves B, Kranz J, Pilatz A, et al. Epidemiology, definition and treatment of complicated urinary tract infections. Nature Reviews Urology. 2020;**17**:586-600. DOI: 10.1038/s41585-020-0362-4

[50] Foxman B. The epidemiology of urinary tract infection. Nature Reviews Urology. 2010;**7**:653-660. DOI: 10.1038/nrurol.2010.190

[51] Haddad JM, Ubertazzi E, Cabrera OS, Medina M, Garcia J, Rodriguez-Colorado S, et al. Latin American consensus on uncomplicated recurrent urinary tract infection—2018. International Urogynecology Journal. 2020;**31**:35-44. DOI: 10.1007/s00192-019-04079-5

[52] Wagenlehner FM, Tandogdu Z, Johansen TEB. An update on classification and management of

urosepsis. Current Opinion in Urology. 2017;**27**:133-137. DOI: 10.1097/mou.0000000000000364

[53] Wagenlehner FME, Naber KG. A new way to prevent urinary tract infections? The Lancet Infectious Diseases. 2017;**17**:467-468. DOI: 10.1016/s1473-3099(17)30107-x

[54] Garrido D, Garrido S, Gutiérrez M, Calvopiña L, Harrison AS, Fuseau M, et al. Clinical characterization and antimicrobial resistance of *Escherichia coli* in pediatric patients with urinary tract infection at a third level hospital of Quito, Ecuador. Boletín Médico del Hospital Infantil de México. 2017;**74**: 265-271. DOI: 10.1016/j.bmhimx.2017.02.004

[55] Jayaweera J, Reyes M. Antimicrobial misuse in pediatric urinary tract infections: Recurrences and renal scarring. Annals of Clinical Microbiology and Antimicrobials. 2018;**17**:27. DOI: 10.1186/s12941-018-0279-4

[56] Conway PH, Cnaan A, Zaoutis T, Henry BV, Grundmeier RW, Keren R. Recurrent urinary tract infections in children: Risk factors and association with prophylactic antimicrobials. Journal of the American Medical Association. 2007;**298**:179-186. DOI: 10.1001/jama.298.2.179

[57] Hoberman A, Charron M, Hickey RW, Baskin M, Kearney DH, Wald ER. Imaging studies after a first febrile urinary tract infection in young children. The New England Journal of Medicine. 2003;**348**:195-202. DOI: 10.1056/NEJMoa021698

[58] Dias CS, Silva JM, Diniz JS, Lima EM, Marciano RC, Lana LG, et al. Risk factors for recurrent urinary tract infections in a cohort of patients with primary vesicoureteral reflux. The Pediatric Infectious Disease Journal. 2010;**29**:139-144. DOI: 10.1097/inf.0b013e3181b8e85f

[59] Zorc JJ, Kiddoo DA, Shaw KN. Diagnosis and management of pediatric urinary tract infections. Clinical Microbiology Reviews. 2005;**18**: 417-422. DOI: 10.1128/cmr.18.2.417-422.2005

[60] Huovinen P. Bacteriotherapy: The time has come. BMJ. 2001;**323**:353-354. DOI: 10.1136/bmj.323.7309.353

[61] Karki T, Truusalu K, Vainumäe I, Mikelsaar M. Antibiotic susceptibility patterns of community- and hospital-acquired *Staphylococcus aureus* and *Escherichia coli* in Estonia. Scandinavian Journal of Infectious Diseases. 2001;**33**: 333-338. DOI: 10.1080/003655401750173904

[62] Worby CJ, Olson BS, Dodson KW, Earl AM, Hultgren SJ. Establishing the role of the gut microbiota in susceptibility to recurrent urinary tract infections. The Journal of Clinical Investigation. 2022;**132**:e158497. DOI: 10.1172/jci158497

[63] Luo Y, Ma Y, Zhao Q, Wang L, Guo L, Ye L, et al. Similarity and divergence of phylogenies, antimicrobial susceptibilities, and virulence factor profiles of *Escherichia coli* isolates causing recurrent urinary tract infections that persist or result from reinfection. Journal of Clinical Microbiology. 2012;**50**:4002-4007. DOI: 10.1128/jcm.02086-12

[64] Jantunen ME, Saxén H, Salo E, Siitonen A. Recurrent urinary tract infections in infancy: Relapses or reinfections? The Journal of Infectious Diseases. 2002;**185**:375-379. DOI: 10.1086/338771

[65] Skjøt-Rasmussen L, Hammerum AM, Jakobsen L, Lester CH, Larsen P, Frimodt-Møller N. Persisting clones of *Escherichia coli* isolates from recurrent urinary tract infection in men and women. Journal of Medical Microbiology. 2011;**60**:550-554. DOI: 10.1099/jmm.0.026963-0

[66] Hunstad DA, Justice SS. Intracellular lifestyles and immune evasion strategies of uropathogenic *Escherichia coli*. Annual Review of Microbiology. 2010;**64**: 203-221. DOI: 10.1146/annurev.micro.112408.134258

[67] Anderson GG, Palermo JJ, Schilling JD, Roth R, Heuser J, Hultgren SJ. Intracellular bacterial biofilm-like pods in urinary tract infections. Science. 2003;**301**:105-107. DOI: 10.1126/science.1084550

[68] Kerrn MB, Struve C, Blom J, Frimodt-Møller N, Krogfelt KA. Intracellular persistence of *Escherichia coli* in urinary bladders from mecillinam-treated mice. Journal of Antimicrobial Chemotherapy. 2005;**55**:383-386. DOI: 10.1093/jac/dki002

[69] Rosen DA, Hooton TM, Stamm WE, Humphrey PA, Hultgren SJ. Detection of intracellular bacterial communities in human urinary tract infection. PLoS Medicine. 2007;**4**:e329. DOI: 10.1371/journal.pmed.0040329

[70] Brown ED, Wright GD. Antibacterial drug discovery in the resistance era. Nature. 2016;**529**:336-343. DOI: 10.1038/nature17042

[71] Khoshnood S, Heidary M, Mirnejad R, Bahramian A, Sedighi M, Mirzaei H. Drug-resistant gram-negative uropathogens: A review. Biomedicine & Pharmacotherapy. 2017;**94**:982-994. DOI: 10.1016/j.biopha.2017.08.006

[72] Pigrau C, Escolà-Vergé L. Infecciones urinarias recurrentes: desde la patogenia a las estrategias de prevención. Medicina Clínica. 2020;**155**: 171-177. DOI: 10.1016/j.medcli.2020.04.026

[73] Carson C, Naber KG. Role of fluoroquinolones in the treatment of serious bacterial urinary tract infections. Drugs. 2004;**64**:1359-1373. DOI: 10.2165/00003495-200464120-00007

[74] Matthew GB, Matthew AM. Persistence of uropathogenic *Escherichia coli* in the face of multiple antibiotics. Antimicrobial Agents and Chemotherapy. 2010;**54**:1855-1863. DOI: 10.1128/AAC.00014-10

[75] Chardavoyne PC, Kasmire KE. Appropriateness of antibiotic prescriptions for urinary tract infections. The Western Journal of Emergency Medicine. 2020;**21**:633-639. DOI: 10.5811/westjem.2020.1.45944

[76] Pratt LA, Kolter R. Genetic analysis of *Escherichia coli* biofilm formation: Roles of flagella, motility, chemotaxis and type I pili. Molecular Microbiology. 1998;**30**:285-293. DOI: 10.1046/j.1365-2958.1998.01061.x

[77] Prigent-Combaret C, Brombacher E, Vidal O, Ambert A, Lejeune P, Landini P, et al. Complex regulatory network controls initial adhesion and biofilm formation in *Escherichia coli* via regulation of the csgD gene. Journal of Bacteriology. 2001;**183**:7213-7223. DOI: 10.1128/jb.183.24.7213-7223.2001

[78] Lewis K. Persister cells and the riddle of biofilm survival. Biochemistry (Moscow). 2005;**70**:267-274. DOI: 10.1007/s10541-005-0111-6

[79] Domka J, Lee J, Bansal T, Wood TK. Temporal gene-expression in *Escherichia*

coli K-12 biofilms. Environmental Microbiology. 2007;**9**:332-346. DOI: 10.1111/j.1462-2920.2006.01143.x

[80] Monds RD, O'Toole GA. The developmental model of microbial biofilms: Ten years of a paradigm up for review. Trends in Microbiology. 2009;**17**: 73-87. DOI: 10.1016/j.tim.2008.11.001

[81] Ferrières L, Aslam SN, Cooper RM, Clarke DJ. The yjbEFGH locus in *Escherichia coli* K-12 is an operon encoding proteins involved in exopolysaccharide production. Microbiology. 2007;**153**:1070-1080. DOI: 10.1099/mic.0.2006/002907-0

[82] Wiles TJ, Kulesus RR, Mulvey MA. Origins and virulence mechanisms of uropathogenic *Escherichia coli*. Experimental and Molecular Pathology. 2008;**85**:11-19. DOI: 10.1016/j.yexmp.2008.03.007

[83] Schwartz DJ, Chen SL, Hultgren SJ, Seed PC. Population dynamics and niche distribution of uropathogenic *Escherichia coli* during acute and chronic urinary tract infection. Infection and Immunity. 2011;**79**(10):4250-4259

[84] Wright KJ, Seed PC, Hultgren SJ. Uropathogenic *Escherichia coli* flagella aid in efficient urinary tract colonization. Infection and Immunity. 2005;**73**: 7657-7668. DOI: 10.1128/iai.73.11.7657-7668.2005

[85] Anderson GG, Goller CC, Justice S, Hultgren SJ, Seed PC. Polysaccharide capsule and sialic acid-mediated regulation promote biofilm-like intracellular bacterial communities during cystitis. Infection and Immunity. 2010;**78**:963-975. DOI: 10.1128/iai.00925-09

[86] AbdelKhalek A, Abutaleb NS, Elmagarmid KA, Seleem MN. Repurposing auranofin as an intestinal decolonizing agent for vancomycin-resistant enterococci. Scientific Reports. 2018;**8**:8353

[87] Jang HI, Eom YB. Repurposing auranofin to combat uropathogenic *Escherichia coli* biofilms. Journal of Applied Microbiology. 2019;**127**(2): 459-471. DOI: 10.1111/jam.14312

[88] Kim Y, Kim S, Cho KH, Lee JH, Lee J. Antibiofilm activities of Cinnamaldehyde analogs against Uropathogenic *Escherichia coli* and *Staphylococcus aureus*. International Journal of Molecular Sciences. 2022; **23**(13):7225. DOI: 10.3390/ijms23137225

[89] Jang M, Cai L, Udeani GO, Slowing KV, Thomas CF, Beecher CW, et al. Cancer chemopreventive activity of resveratrol, a natural product derived from grapes. Science. 1997;**275**:218-220. DOI: 10.1126/science.275.5297.218

[90] Cottart CH, Nivet-Antoine V, Laguillier-Morizot C, Beaudeux JL. Resveratrol bioavailability and toxicity in humans. Molecular Nutrition & Food Research. 2010;**54**:7-16. DOI: 10.1002/mnfr.200900437

[91] Oh M, Lee J-H, Bae SY, Seok JH, Kim S, Chung YB, et al. Protective effects of red wine and resveratrol for foodborne virus surrogates. Food Control. 2015;**47**:502-509. DOI: 10.1016/j.foodcont.2014.07.056

[92] Ma DSL, Tan LT, Chan KG, Yap WH, Pusparajah P, Chuah LH, et al. Resveratrol-potential antibacterial agent against foodborne pathogens. Frontiers in Pharmacology. 2018;**9**:102. DOI: 10.3389/fphar.2018.00102

[93] Vestergaard M, Ingmer H. Antibacterial and antifungal properties of resveratrol. International Journal of

Antimicrobial Agents. 2019;**53**:716-723. DOI: 10.1016/j.ijantimicag.2019.02.015

[94] Lee JH, Kim YG, Raorane CJ, Ryu SY, Shim JJ, Lee J. The anti-biofilm and anti-virulence activities of *trans*-resveratrol and oxyresveratrol against uropathogenic *Escherichia coli*. Biofouling. 2019;**35**(7):758-767. DOI: 10.1080/08927014.2019.1657418

[95] Vasudevan S, Thamil Selvan G, Bhaskaran S, Hari N, Solomon AP. Reciprocal cooperation of type a Procyanidin and nitrofurantoin against multi-drug resistant (MDR) UPEC: A pH-dependent study. Frontiers in Cellular and Infection Microbiology. 2020;**10**:421. DOI: 10.3389/fcimb.2020.00421

[96] Thänert R, Reske KA, Hink T, Wallace MA, Wang B, Schwartz DJ, et al. Comparative genomics of antibiotic-resistant uropathogens implicates three routes for recurrence of urinary tract infections. MBio. 2019;**10**:e01977-e01919. DOI: 10.1128/mBio.01977-19

[97] Lamm ME. Interaction of antigens and antibodies at mucosal surfaces. Annual Review of Microbiology. 1997;**51**:311-340. DOI: 10.1146/annurev.micro.51.1.311

[98] Levine MM. Immunization against bacterial diseases of the intestine. Journal of Pediatric Gastroenterology and Nutrition. 2000;**31**:336-355. DOI: 10.1097/00005176-200010000-00003

[99] Kochiashvili D, Khuskivadze A, Kochiashvili G, Koberidze G, Kvakhajelidze V. Role of the bacterial vaccine Solco-Urovac® in treatment and prevention of recurrent urinary tract infections of bacterial origin. Georgian Medical News. 2014;**231**:11-16

[100] Hopkins WJ, Elkahwaji J, Beierle LM, Leverson GE, Uehling DT. Vaginal mucosal vaccine for recurrent urinary tract infections in women: Results of a phase 2 clinical trial. The Journal of Urology. 2007;**177**:1349-1353; quiz 1591. DOI: 10.1016/j.juro.2006.11.093

[101] Nestler S, Peschel C, Horstmann AH, Vahlensieck W, Fabry W, Neisius A. Prospective multicentre randomized double-blind placebo-controlled parallel group study on the efficacy and tolerability of StroVac® in patients with recurrent symptomatic uncomplicated bacterial urinary tract infections. International Urology and Nephrology. 2022;**54**:1-8

[102] Bauer HW, Alloussi S, Egger G, Blümlein HM, Cozma G, Schulman CC. A long-term, multicenter, double-blind study of an *Escherichia coli* extract (OM-89) in female patients with recurrent urinary tract infections. European Urology. 2005;**47**:542-548; discussion 548. DOI: 10.1016/j.eururo.2004.12.009

[103] Huttner A, Gambillara V. The development and early clinical testing of the ExPEC4V conjugate vaccine against uropathogenic *Escherichia coli*. Clinical Microbiology and Infection. 2018; **24**(10):1046-1050

[104] Huttner A, Hatz C, van den Dobbelsteen G, Abbanat D, Hornacek A, Frölich R, et al. Safety, immunogenicity, and preliminary clinical efficacy of a vaccine against extraintestinal pathogenic *Escherichia coli* in women with a history of recurrent urinary tract infection: A randomised, single-blind, placebo-controlled phase 1b trial. The Lancet Infectious Diseases. 2017;**17**(5):528-537

[105] Nickel JC, Saz-Leal P, Doiron RC. Could sublingual vaccination be a viable

option for the prevention of recurrent urinary tract infection in Canada? A systematic review of the current literature and plans for the future. Canadian Urological Association Journal. 2020;**14**(8):281

[106] Billips BK, Yaggie RE, Cashy JP, Schaeffer AJ, Klumpp DJ. A live-attenuated vaccine for the treatment of urinary tract infection by uropathogenic *Escherichia coli*. The Journal of Infectious Diseases. 2009;**200**:263-272. DOI: 10.1086/599839

[107] Brumbaugh AR, Mobley HL. Preventing urinary tract infection: Progress toward an effective *Escherichia coli* vaccine. Expert Review of Vaccines. 2012;**11**:663-676. DOI: 10.1586/erv.12.36

[108] Connell I, Agace W, Klemm P, Schembri M, Mărild S, Svanborg C. Type 1 fimbrial expression enhances *Escherichia coli* virulence for the urinary tract. Proceedings of the National Academy of Sciences of the United States of America. 1996;**93**:9827-9832. DOI: 10.1073/pnas.93.18.9827

[109] Norinder BS, Köves B, Yadav M, Brauner A, Svanborg C. Do *Escherichia coli* strains causing acute cystitis have a distinct virulence repertoire? Microbial Pathogenesis. 2012;**52**:10-16. DOI: 10.1016/j.micpath.2011.08.005

[110] Cordeiro MA, Werle CH, Milanez GP, Yano T. Curli fimbria: An *Escherichia coli* adhesin associated with human cystitis. Brazilian Journal of Microbiology. 2016;**47**:414-416. DOI: 10.1016/j.bjm.2016.01.024

[111] Manning SD, Zhang L, Foxman B, Spindler A, Tallman P, Marrs CF. Prevalence of known P-fimbrial G alleles in *Escherichia coli* and identification of a new adhesin class. Clinical and Diagnostic Laboratory Immunology. 2001;**8**:637-640. DOI: 10.1128/cdli.8.3.637-640.2001

[112] Thankavel K, Madison B, Ikeda T, Malaviya R, Shah AH, Arumugam PM, et al. Localization of a domain in the FimH adhesin of *Escherichia coli* type 1 fimbriae capable of receptor recognition and use of a domain-specific antibody to confer protection against experimental urinary tract infection. The Journal of Clinical Investigation. 1997;**100**: 1123-1136. DOI: 10.1172/jci119623

[113] Langermann S, Ballou WR Jr. Vaccination utilizing the FimCH complex as a strategy to prevent *Escherichia coli* urinary tract infections. The Journal of Infectious Diseases. 2001; **183**:S84-S86. DOI: 10.1086/318857

[114] Langermann S, Ballou WR. Development of a recombinant FIMCH vaccine for urinary tract infections. In: Atala A, Slade D, editors. Bladder Disease, Part a: Research Concepts and Clinical Applications. Boston, MA: Springer US; 2003. pp. 635-653

[115] Habibi M, Asadi Karam MR, Shokrgozar MA, Oloomi M, Jafari A, Bouzari S. Intranasal immunization with fusion protein MrpH·FimH and MPL adjuvant confers protection against urinary tract infections caused by uropathogenic *Escherichia coli* and *Proteus mirabilis*. Molecular Immunology. 2015;**64**:285-294. DOI: 10.1016/j.molimm.2014.12.008

[116] Fischer H, Yamamoto M, Akira S, Beutler B, Svanborg C. Mechanism of pathogen-specific TLR4 activation in the mucosa: Fimbriae, recognition receptors and adaptor protein selection. European Journal of Immunology. 2006;**36**: 267-277. DOI: 10.1002/eji.200535149

[117] Samuelsson P, Hang L, Wullt B, Irjala H, Svanborg C. Toll-like receptor 4

expression and cytokine responses in the human urinary tract mucosa. Infection and Immunity. 2004;**72**:3179-3186. DOI: 10.1128/iai.72.6.3179-3186.2004

[118] Lane MC, Mobley HLT. Role of P-fimbrial-mediated adherence in pyelonephritis and persistence of uropathogenic *Escherichia coli* (UPEC) in the mammalian kidney. Kidney International. 2007;**72**:19-25. DOI: 10.1038/sj.ki.5002230

[119] Frendéus B, Wachtler C, Hedlund M, Fischer H, Samuelsson P, Svensson M, et al. *Escherichia coli P. fimbriae* utilize the toll-like receptor 4 pathway for cell activation. Molecular Microbiology. 2001;**40**:37-51. DOI: 10.1046/j.1365-2958.2001.02361.x

[120] Pecha B, Low D, O'Hanley P. Gal-gal pili vaccines prevent pyelonephritis by piliated *Escherichia coli* in a murine model. Single-component gal-gal pili vaccines prevent pyelonephritis by homologous and heterologous piliated E. coli strains. The Journal of Clinical Investigation. 1989;**83**:2102-2108. DOI: 10.1172/jci114123

[121] Bian Z, Brauner A, Li Y, Normark S. Expression of and cytokine activation by *Escherichia coli* curli fibers in human sepsis. The Journal of Infectious Diseases. 2000;**181**:602-612. DOI: 10.1086/315233

[122] Tükel C, Nishimori JH, Wilson RP, Winter MG, Keestra AM, van Putten JP, et al. Toll-like receptors 1 and 2 cooperatively mediate immune responses to curli, a common amyloid from enterobacterial biofilms. Cellular Microbiology. 2010;**12**:1495-1505. DOI: 10.1111/j.1462-5822.2010.01485.x

[123] Bian Z, Yan Z-Q, Hansson GK, Thorén P, Normark S. Activation of inducible nitric oxide synthase/nitric oxide by curli fibers leads to a fall in blood pressure during systemic *Escherichia coli* infection in mice. The Journal of Infectious Diseases. 2001;**183**: 612-619. DOI: 10.1086/318528

[124] Rapsinski GJ, Wynosky-Dolfi MA, Oppong GO, Tursi SA, Wilson RP, Brodsky IE, et al. Toll-like receptor 2 and NLRP3 cooperate to recognize a functional bacterial amyloid, curli. Infection and Immunity. 2015;**83**: 693-701. DOI: 10.1128/iai.02370-14